RENAL DIET COOKBOOK FOR BEGINNERS

Nourishing Fragile Kidneys With A Collection Of Quick, Delicious And Healthy Low Sodium, Potassium, and Phosphorus Recipes

Kimberly Mullins

I just wanted to drop you a quick note to say a huge thank you for buying my book. Your support really means a lot to me, and I hope you find the recipes helpful and enjoyable.

Disclaimer:

The information provided in this communication is for general informational
 only. It should not be considered as professional, legal, medical, or financial advice. You are encouraged to seek advice and confirmation from qualified experts or professionals before making any decisions or taking actions based on the content provided here. We do not guarantee the accuracy, completeness, or suitability of the information and shall not be liable for any errors, omissions, or damages arising from its use. Any reliance you place on this information is strictly at your own risk. This communication does not create a professional-client relationship. Any views or opinions expressed here are solely those of the individual author and do not necessarily represent the views of any organization or entity. We reserve the right to modify, update, or remove content at any time without notice. By continuing to read or interact with this content, you agree to these terms and conditions.

ABOUT THE AUTHOR

Kimberly Mullins is a renowned chef and dedicated dietitian with a passion for promoting healthy eating and lifestyle choices. With a culinary flair and a deep understanding of nutrition, she has made it her mission to inspire individuals and families to live happier, healthier lives through the food they consume.

As a chef, Kimberly's expertise lies in crafting delectable dishes that not only tantalize the taste buds but also nourish the body. Her culinary creations seamlessly blend flavors, textures, and ingredients to make wholesome meals that cater to a wide range of dietary preferences and restrictions.

Simultaneously, Kimberly's background as a dietitian empowers her to provide sound nutritional advice and guidance. She understands the intricate relationship between food and well-being and strives to educate others on making informed choices for optimal health.

Beyond her professional pursuits, Kimberly is a loving wife and a devoted mother of two. Her own family serves as the cornerstone of her commitment to health and wellness, driving her to explore creative ways to make nutritious eating an enjoyable and integral part of daily life.

Kimberly Mullins' journey in the culinary and dietary world has led her to become a trusted source of expertise, helping countless individuals and families embrace a lifestyle that prioritizes health, balance, and deliciousness. Through her writing and culinary creations, she continues to inspire and guide others toward a more vibrant and wholesome way of living.

TABLE OF CONTENTS

INTRODUCTION

Hey there! I'm thrilled to have you join me on this journey as we unravel the mysteries of kidney health and nutrition together.

Okay, let's get real for a moment. Our kidneys? They're like the secret super heroes of our bodies, quietly working behind the scenes to keep us ticking along smoothly. But what occurs if there's a hiccup along the way? That's where things get tricky.

So, picture this: You've just found out you or someone you care about has kidney issues. It's scary, right? I get it. But hey, guess what? You're not alone, my friend. And that's why we're here—together, to figure this out and take charge of our health like the champs we are.

Now, I won't sugarcoat it—navigating the world of kidney-friendly diets can feel like diving headfirst into a bowl of alphabet soup. Phosphorus? Potassium? Sodium? Say what now? It's enough to make your head spin!

But fear not, my fellow kidney warriors, because that's where this book swoops in to save the day. We're gonna break it down, step by step, in a way that even your grandma could understand. No fancy medical jargon here—just good old-fashioned advice served up with a side of heart and humor.

Throughout these pages, we're gonna explore everything from the basics of kidney health to the nitty-gritty details of crafting a kidney-friendly plate that's as delicious as it is nutritious. Life's too short to eat bland food all the time, am I right?

So, grab a cozy spot, pour yourself a cup of your favorite beverage (water's a good choice!), and let's dive in. Together, we're gonna learn, laugh, and maybe even shed a tear or two along the way. But most importantly, we're gonna take control of our health and show those kidneys some serious love.

Because hey, who says a kidney-friendly diet can't be fun? Not us!

CHAPTER 1: THE RENAL DIET FUNDAMENTAL

What is a renal diet??

It's a diet that's specifically designed to support optimal kidney function and manage the symptoms of kidney disease. It's like a customized meal plan that takes into account the unique needs of your kidneys and helps ensure you're getting the right balance of nutrients to keep them happy and healthy.

Now, you might be wondering why a renal diet is necessary in the first place. Well, here's the deal: When your kidneys aren't working as well as they should, certain nutrients can build up in your blood and cause all sorts of problems. Things like sodium, potassium, phosphorus, and protein can become a bit of a balancing act, and that's where a renal diet comes in.

The goal of a renal diet is twofold: to help reduce the workload on your kidneys by limiting the intake of certain nutrients that can be hard for them to process, and to provide you with the nutrients your body needs to stay healthy and strong. It's all about finding the right balance that supports kidney function while still allowing you to enjoy a varied and delicious diet.

Now, let's break it down a bit further. A renal diet typically involves:

1. Limiting Sodium: Sodium can cause your body to retain fluid and raise your blood pressure, putting extra strain on your kidneys. So, cutting back on salty foods and processed snacks is often a key component of a renal diet.

2. Managing Potassium: Potassium is important for nerve and muscle function, but too much of it can be harmful if your kidneys aren't able to regulate it properly. So, keeping an eye on your potassium intake—especially if you have kidney disease—is crucial.

3. Watching Phosphorus: Phosphorus is found in many foods, especially protein-rich ones, and can build up in your blood if your kidneys aren't able to remove it efficiently. So, limiting phosphorus-rich foods like dairy, nuts, and processed meats is often recommended.

4. Balancing Protein: Protein is essential for building and repairing tissues in your body, but eating too much of it can put extra strain on your kidneys. So, finding the right balance of high-quality protein sources while still meeting your nutritional needs is key.

In addition to these key nutrients, a renal diet may also involve other dietary considerations like managing fluid intake, controlling blood sugar levels (especially if you have diabetes), and making sure you're getting enough vitamins and minerals to support overall health.

Benefits of a renal diet

When it comes to managing kidney health, a renal diet aims to achieve a few key objectives:

1. Supporting Optimal Kidney Function: The primary goal of a renal diet is to support the optimal function of your kidneys. By providing your body with the right balance of nutrients and minimizing the intake of substances that can put extra strain on your kidneys, a renal diet helps ensure that your kidneys can do their job effectively and efficiently.

2. Managing Symptoms of Kidney Disease: For individuals with kidney disease, a renal diet can help manage the symptoms and complications associated with impaired kidney function. By controlling factors like blood pressure, fluid balance, and electrolyte levels, a renal diet can help reduce the risk of complications like fluid retention, high blood pressure, and electrolyte imbalances.

3. Preventing Further Damage to the Kidneys: In some cases, following a renal diet can help slow the progression of kidney disease and prevent further damage to the kidneys. By reducing the workload on your kidneys and minimizing the build-up of harmful substances in your blood, a renal diet can help preserve kidney function and delay the need for more intensive medical procedures like kidney transplants or dialysis.

Now, let's talk about the benefits of following a renal diet. Here are just a few reasons why embracing kidney-friendly eating can have a positive impact on your overall health and well-being:

1. Improved Kidney Function: By providing your body with the nutrients it needs to support kidney function and minimizing the intake of substances that can harm your kidneys, a renal diet can help improve overall kidney health and function.

2. Better Management of Symptoms: Following a renal diet can help manage the symptoms and complications associated with kidney disease, such as high blood pressure, fluid retention, and electrolyte imbalances. This can lead to improved quality of life and reduced risk of complications.

3. Reduced Risk of Complications: By controlling factors like blood pressure, fluid balance, and electrolyte levels, a renal diet can help reduce the risk of complications like heart disease, stroke, and kidney failure.

4. Enhanced Overall Health: Embracing kidney-friendly eating often involves adopting a diet that's rich in fruits, vegetables, whole grains, and lean proteins, while limiting processed foods, sodium, and unhealthy fats. This can lead to improved overall health, including better control of blood sugar levels, lower cholesterol, and healthier weight management.

Remember, embracing kidney-friendly eating isn't just about what you can't eat—it's about nourishing your body and supporting your kidneys to help you live your healthiest, happiest life possible.

CHAPTER 2: NUTRIENTS AND THEIR IMPACT

Sodium

When it comes to kidney health, managing sodium intake is crucial. Sodium, an essential mineral found in salt, plays a vital role in maintaining fluid balance, transmitting nerve impulses, and supporting muscle function. However, for individuals with kidney issues, excessive sodium intake can exacerbate problems and lead to serious complications.

Why Sodium Matters in Kidney Health?

• **Fluid Balance:** One of the kidneys' primary functions is to regulate the body's fluid balance. Water and sodium are tightly related; water always follows sodium. High sodium levels can cause the body to retain excess fluid, increasing the burden on the kidneys and potentially leading to swelling (edema), high blood pressure, and heart issues.

• **Blood Pressure Regulation:** The effects of sodium on blood pressure are substantial.
High sodium intake can cause an increase in blood pressure, which is a major risk factor for both chronic kidney disease (CKD) and heart disease. When the kidneys are already compromised, managing blood pressure becomes even more critical to prevent further damage.

• **Electrolyte Balance:** The kidneys also help maintain the balance of electrolytes, including sodium, potassium, and chloride, which are essential for many bodily functions. Disrupting this balance can lead to complications, particularly for those with kidney disease.

Strategies for Reducing Sodium Intake

• **Read Food Labels:** Sodium can be hidden in many processed and packaged foods. Always check the nutrition labels for sodium content and choose low-sodium or sodium-free options when possible.

• **Cook at Home:** You can regulate how much salt is in your food by making meals at home. Use fresh ingredients and avoid pre-packaged seasonings and sauces that are often high in sodium.

• **Use Herbs and Spices:** Instead of relying on salt to flavor your food, experiment with herbs, spices, and other salt-free seasonings. Garlic, lemon juice, vinegar, and pepper can add a lot of flavor without the added sodium.

• **Limit Processed Foods**: Processed foods, including canned soups, frozen meals, and snack foods, are often high in sodium. Choose whole fresh meals, whenever possible.

• **Rinse Canned Foods:** If you use canned vegetables or beans, rinse them thoroughly under water to remove some of the excess sodium.

• **Choose Low-Sodium Alternatives:** Many products come in low-sodium versions, such as broths, soups, and sauces. Look for these alternatives to reduce your sodium intake.

• **Be Mindful of Restaurant Meals:** Dining out can be tricky since restaurant meals often contain high amounts of sodium. Ask for nutritional information when available, request that your food be prepared without added salt, and choose dishes that are steamed, grilled, or baked.

<u>**Note**</u>
Aim to consume less than 2,000 milligrams (mg) of sodium per day, or lower if recommended by your healthcare provider.

Phosphorus

Phosphorus is an essential mineral that plays a crucial role in many bodily functions, including the formation of bones and teeth, energy production, and the regulation of various biochemical reactions. However, for individuals with kidney disease, managing phosphorus intake is vital to prevent complications and support overall health.

The Role of Phosphorus in the Body

• **Bone Health:** Phosphorus works closely with calcium to build and maintain strong bones and teeth. About 85% of the phosphorus in the human body is found in bones and teeth.

• **Energy Production:** Phosphorus is a component of ATP (adenosine triphosphate), which is the primary energy carrier in cells. This makes it essential for energy production and storage.

• **Cell Function:** Phosphorus plays a key role in the structure and function of cell membranes, DNA, and RNA. It is involved in many cellular processes, including the regulation of acid-base balance.

Why Phosphorus Management is Crucial in Kidney Health

For healthy individuals, the kidneys regulate the amount of phosphorus in the blood by filtering out excess phosphorus and excreting it through urine. However, when the kidneys are not functioning properly, they can't remove phosphorus efficiently, leading to high levels in the blood—a condition known as hyperphosphatemia.

Hyperphosphatemia
This condition occurs when there is too much phosphorus in the blood. High phosphorus levels can lead to several health issues, including:

1. **Bone and Joint Problems:** Excess phosphorus can pull calcium from the bones, weakening them and increasing the risk of fractures and joint pain. This can also lead to a condition called renal osteodystrophy, a type of bone disease that occurs in people with kidney disease.

2. **Vascular Calcification:** High phosphorus levels can cause calcium deposits to form in blood vessels, heart, and other soft tissues. This can lead to cardiovascular diseases, which are a major cause of morbidity and mortality in individuals with kidney disease.

3. Parathyroid Hormone (PTH) Imbalance: Elevated phosphorus levels can trigger the release of PTH, leading to secondary hyperparathyroidism. This condition can cause further bone loss and calcium imbalances.

Strategies for Managing Phosphorus Intake

Managing phosphorus intake involves dietary adjustments, monitoring, and sometimes medication. Here are key strategies:

1. Choose Low-Phosphorus Foods: Certain foods are high in phosphorus, such as dairy products, meat, fish, poultry, nuts, seeds, beans, and whole grains. Opt for lower-phosphorus options like fresh fruits, vegetables, rice, and refined grains.

2. Limit Processed Foods: Many processed and packaged foods contain added phosphorus in the form of phosphate additives. These additives are easily absorbed by the body and can significantly increase phosphorus levels. Check food labels for ingredients like "phosphate," "phosphoric acid," and "sodium phosphate."

3. Use Phosphate Binders: If dietary restrictions are not enough to control phosphorus levels, your healthcare provider may prescribe phosphate binders. These medications help bind phosphorus in the gut, reducing its absorption and lowering blood phosphorus levels. Always take phosphate binders as directed.

4. Balance Calcium and Vitamin D Intake: Calcium and vitamin D are important for bone health and can help counteract the effects of high phosphorus levels. Your healthcare provider may recommend supplements or dietary adjustments to ensure you're getting the right balance.

5. Monitor Portion Sizes: Even foods that are moderate in phosphorus can contribute to high levels if consumed in large quantities. Be mindful of portion sizes to help keep phosphorus intake within recommended limits.

Practical Tips for Daily Phosphorus Management

- **Read Food Labels:** Look for phosphorus content on nutrition labels and avoid foods with phosphate additives.

- **Cook at Home:** Preparing meals at home allows you to control the ingredients and avoid high-phosphorus additives found in many processed foods.
- **Soak and Cook Legumes:** If you consume legumes, soaking them overnight and cooking them in fresh water can help reduce their phosphorus content.

Protein

Protein is an essential macronutrient that plays a crucial role in building and repairing tissues, supporting immune function, and serving as a vital component of enzymes and hormones. However, for individuals with kidney disease, managing protein intake is important to support kidney function and overall health.

Why Protein Management is Crucial in Kidney Health

For individuals with healthy kidneys, consuming adequate protein is vital for maintaining muscle mass and overall health. However, for those with kidney disease, the kidneys' ability to filter waste products from protein metabolism, such as urea, is impaired. This can lead to an accumulation of waste products in the blood, which can exacerbate kidney damage and lead to other health complications.

Excessive Protein Intake: High protein intake can increase the workload on the kidneys, accelerating the progression of kidney damage and worsening kidney function. It can also lead to an increase in waste products like urea and creatinine in the blood.

Insufficient Protein Intake: On the other hand, consuming too little protein can lead to muscle wasting, weakened immune function, and overall poor health. Therefore, finding the right balance of protein intake is essential for individuals with kidney disease.

Goals of Protein Management

The primary goals of managing protein intake in a renal diet are:

1. Minimizing Kidney Workload: Reducing the amount of waste products the kidneys need to filter helps lessen the burden on these vital organs.

2. Maintaining Muscle Mass: Ensuring adequate protein intake to prevent muscle wasting and maintain overall strength and function.

3. Supporting Overall Health: Balancing protein intake to support immune function, energy levels, and overall well-being.

Strategies for Managing Protein Intake

Finding the right balance of protein involves dietary adjustments, monitoring, and sometimes working with a healthcare provider or dietitian. Here are key strategies:

1. Determine Protein Needs: Protein needs can vary based on the stage of kidney disease, body weight, age, and overall health. Work with a healthcare provider to determine the appropriate amount of protein for your specific situation.

2. Choose High-Quality Protein Sources: Focus on high-quality protein sources that provide essential amino acids. Good options include lean meats, poultry, fish, eggs, dairy products, beans, and legumes. Plant-based proteins, such as tofu and tempeh, can also be excellent choices.

3. Monitor Portion Sizes: Even high-quality proteins should be consumed in appropriate portions to avoid excessive intake. Be mindful of portion sizes and spread protein intake evenly throughout the day.

4. Combine Protein Sources: Combining different protein sources can help ensure you get a variety of essential amino acids. For example, pairing beans with rice or whole grains can provide a complete protein profile.

5. Limit Processed and High-Phosphorus Proteins: Processed meats, such as deli meats, sausages, and bacon, often contain high levels of phosphorus and sodium, which can be harmful for kidney health. Opt for fresh, unprocessed protein sources instead.

Potassium

Why Potassium Matters in Kidney Health

• **Muscle and Nerve Function:** Potassium is necessary for the proper function of muscles and nerves. It helps regulate muscle contractions, including the vital contraction of the heart muscle, and supports the transmission of nerve impulses.

• **Fluid and Electrolyte Balance:** Potassium works closely with sodium to maintain the body's fluid balance and ensure that cells, tissues, and organs function properly. Maintaining the right balance of these electrolytes is crucial for overall health.

• **Heart Health:** Potassium plays a key role in maintaining a regular heart rhythm. Too much or too little potassium can cause dangerous changes in heart rate, potentially leading to arrhythmias or other cardiac issues.

For individuals with healthy kidneys, maintaining potassium balance is relatively straightforward, as the kidneys efficiently filter out excess potassium through urine. However, for those with kidney disease or compromised kidney function, this process can be impaired, leading to the risk of hyperkalemia (high potassium levels) or hypokalemia (low potassium levels).

For individuals with kidney issues, the primary goals of potassium management are:

1. Maintaining Safe Potassium Levels: Ensuring that blood potassium levels remain within a safe range to prevent the risks associated with hyperkalemia and hypokalemia.

2. Supporting Overall Health: Balancing potassium intake helps support overall health by ensuring proper muscle and nerve function, fluid balance, and heart health.

3. Preventing Complications: Effective potassium management can reduce the risk of complications such as cardiac arrhythmias and muscle weakness

CHAPTER 3: BUILDING A FRIENDLY KIDNEY PLATE

Portion Control

Portion control and understanding serving sizes are essential components of a renal diet. For individuals with kidney disease, managing the intake of certain nutrients like sodium, potassium, phosphorus, and protein is crucial to support kidney function and prevent complications. Here's a comprehensive guide on portion control and serving sizes to help you navigate your renal diet effectively:

Practical Tips for Portion Control

• **Use Smaller Plates and Bowls:** Smaller dishware can make portions appear larger, helping to trick your brain into feeling satisfied with less food.

• **Measure and Weigh Food:** Use measuring cups, spoons, and a kitchen scale to accurately measure portions, especially when starting to learn about serving sizes.

• **Read Food Labels:** Food labels provide serving size information and nutritional content, which can guide portion control. Take note of how many servings each container holds

• **Plan Meals and Snacks**: Pre-planning meals and snacks can help manage portion sizes and avoid compulsive eating. Portion out snacks into individual servings rather than eating from a large container.

• **Eat Mindfully:** Slow down and savor each bite. Eating mindfully can help you recognize when you're full and prevent overeating.

• **Be Consistent with Portions:** Keep portions consistent to maintain balanced nutrient intake. Adjust portions if you notice changes in your weight or health status, and consult your dietitian for guidance.

High-Sodium Foods to Avoid

Processed and Packaged Foods
- **Canned Soups and Stews**: These often contain high levels of sodium as preservatives and flavor enhancers.
- **Instant Noodles: Pre**-packaged noodle soups usually have high sodium content.
- **Frozen Meals:** Many frozen dinners, especially those with sauces or gravies, are high in sodium.
- **Snack Foods:** Potato chips, pretzels, and salted nuts are typically high in sodium.

Cured and Processed Meats
- **Deli Meats:** Ham, salami, bologna, and other processed deli meats are often loaded with sodium.
- **Bacon and Sausages**: Both fresh and pre-cooked varieties usually contain high amounts of sodium.
- **Hot Dogs:** These are typically high in sodium and preservatives.

Condiments and Sauces
- **Soy Sauce:** Even low-sodium versions can still be quite high in sodium.
- **Ketchup**: Contains added salt and sugar.
- **Barbecue Sauce:** Often contains high levels of sodium and sugar.
- **Salad Dressings**: Many commercial dressings, especially creamy ones, are high in sodium.

Cheese and Dairy Products
- **Processed Cheeses**: Cheese slices, cheese spreads, and pre-packaged cheese products usually contain a lot of sodium.
- **Feta and Blue Cheese:** These varieties are often higher in sodium compared to others.

Breads and Baked Goods
- **Commercial Breads:** Many types of store-bought bread and rolls contain added salt.

- **Biscuits and Muffins**: Especially those from fast-food restaurants or pre-packaged versions.

<u>**Restaurant and Fast Foods**</u>
- **Food Burgers and Sandwiches**: Often contain high sodium levels in the meat, cheese, and condiments.
- **Pizza:** Both the crust and toppings can have a high sodium content.

Sodium Healthier Alternatives

- **Fresh Vegetables:** Opt for fresh vegetables and prepare them without added salt.
- **Frozen Vegetables**: Choose those without added sauces or seasoning.

- **Low-Sodium Canned Vegetables** Rinse them under water to remove excess sodium.
- **Low-Sodium Soups:** Choose brands that offer low-sodium options or make homemade soup to control the salt content.

- **Fresh Meat, Poultry, and Fish:** Choose fresh over processed. Prepare them with herbs and spices instead of salt.
- **Eggs**: A good low-sodium protein option when prepared without added salt.

- **Herbs and Spices**: Use fresh or dried herbs, garlic, onion powder, and spices like pepper, cumin, and paprika.
- **Lemon Juice and Vinegar**: Add flavor sodium.
- **Low-Sodium Sauces:** Look for low-sodium soy sauce or make your own dressings and marinades.

- **Fresh Cheese:** Mozzarella, Swiss, and goat cheese tend to have lower sodium levels.
- **Unsweetened Dairy Alternatives:** Almond milk, rice milk, or coconut milk without added sodium.

- **Whole Grain Bread:** Look for brands with lower sodium or bake your own at home.
- **Oats and Quinoa:** Naturally low in sodium and a good base for meals.
- **Unsalted Nuts and Seeds:** A healthier option compared to salted versions.

- **Water**
- **Unsweetened Teas and Coffee**

High-Potassium Foods to Avoid

<u>Fruits</u>
- Bananas
- Oranges and Orange Juice
- Avocados
- Cantaloupe and Honeydew
- Dried Fruits
- Kiwi
- Mango
- Pear

<u>Vegetables</u>
- Potatoes White and sweet potatoes, especially with the skin.
- Tomatoes Fresh, canned, sauce, and paste.
- Spinach Especially when cooked.
- Beet Greens
- Artichokes
- Winter Squash Such as acorn, butternut, and pumpkin.

<u>Dairy Products</u>
- Milk and Yogurt
- Cheese Some cheeses have moderate to high potassium levels.
- Ice Cream Contains potassium, especially if it has added chocolate or nuts.

<u>Legumes and Nuts</u>
- Black beans, lentils, and kidney beans
- Almonds, peanuts, and other nuts
- Pumpkin and sunflower seeds.

<u>Grains</u>
- Brown rice, quinoa, and whole wheat products have higher potassium than their refined counterparts.

<u>**Fish and Meats**</u>
- Salmon, halibut, and tuna
- Beef, pork, and chicken in large portions can contribute to higher potassium intake.

<u>**Beverages**</u>
- Sports Drinks
- Coffee Especially if consumed in large quantities.

Lower-Potassium and Phosphorus Substitutes

Fruits
- Apples
- Berries: Strawberries, blueberries, raspberries, and blackberries.
- Grapes
 - Peaches and Plums:
- Pineapple
- Cranberries

Vegetables
- Cauliflower Fresh or cooked.
- Cabbage Fresh or cooked.
- Cucumbers Fresh, in salads, or as pickles (low-sodium).
- Green Beans
- Bell Peppers
- Lettuce: All types, used in salads or sandwiches.
- Onions

Dairy Alternatives
- Rice Milk Unsweetened versions.
- Almond Milk Unsweetened and lower potassium versions.
- Non-Dairy Creamer Low-potassium options for coffee or tea.

Protein Sources
- Egg Whites
- Chicken Breast Skinless, grilled, baked, or boiled.
- Turkey Breast Skinless, grilled, baked, or boiled.
- Fish Cod, tilapia, and tuna (low-sodium canned or fresh).
- Tofu is a good plant-based protein option, lower in potassium than beans.

Grains and Starches
- White Rice
- Pasta
- White Bread
- Tortillas Corn or flour, low-sodium versions.
- Unsalted Popcorn.

Healthy Fats
- Olive Oil
- Canola Oil.
- Unsalted Butter or Margarine In moderation.

Beverages
- Clear Sodas Like ginger ale or lemon-lime soda, in moderation.
- Coffee and Tea Without added potassium-containing creamers, in moderation.

For high-potassium vegetables like potatoes, leaching can reduce potassium content. Cut the vegetable into small pieces, soak in water for a few hours, rinse, and cook in freshwater.

Phosphorus-Rich Foods to Avoid

- Milk.
- Hard Cheese (cheddar and Parmesan)
- Yogurt
- Ice Cream High in phosphorus, especially with added nuts or chocolate.

- Organ Meats: Liver, kidneys, and other organ meats are very high in phosphorus.
- Processed Meats: Bacon, hot dogs, sausages, and deli meats.
- Fish: Salmon, tuna, and other fatty fish.
- Shellfish: Shrimp, crab, and other shellfish.

- Brown rice, whole wheat bread, and oatmeal are higher in phosphorus than their refined counterparts.
- Bran Cereals
- Almonds, peanuts, sunflower seeds, and others.

- Lentils, chickpeas, and black beans.
- Tofu, edamame, and soy milk.

- Colas
- Beer
- Dark-Colored Sodas
- Fast Food Burgers, pizza, and fried foods.
- Frozen Meals Especially those with sauces and gravies.
- Packaged Snacks: Potato chips, pretzels, and microwave popcorn with added phosphorus.

- Chocolate
- Pancake and muffin mixes.

BREAKFAST RECIPES

English Muffin with Hummus & Veggies

Prep Time: 5 minutes | Cook Time: 5 minutes | Serves: 1

Ingredients:
- 1 whole-grain English muffin, split and lightly toasted (low-sodium)
- 2 tablespoons homemade or store-bought low-sodium hummus
- 1/4 cup thinly sliced cucumber
- 1/4 cup thinly sliced bell pepper (any color)
- One tablespoon of optional fresh parsley, chopped for garnish)
- Black pepper to taste

Instructions:
1. Lightly toast the whole-grain English muffin in a toaster until just golden brown.

2. Once toasted, spread a modest amount of low-sodium hummus evenly onto each English muffin half.

3. Arrange the thinly sliced cucumber and bell pepper on top of the hummus-covered English muffin halves.

4. Sprinkle a dash of black pepper over the veggies for added flavor.

5. For a touch of freshness and flavor, sprinkle chopped parsley over the veggies.

Cooking Tips:
- Use homemade hummus made with soaked chickpeas to further reduce sodium content.
- Rinse vegetables under cold water to remove excess potassium.
- Pair with a side of low-phosphorus, low-potassium protein such as egg whites or tofu for added sustenance.

Nutritional Information (per serving):
- Calories: 200
- Protein: 5g
- Carbohydrates: 35g
- Fiber: 8g
- Sodium: 80mg
- Potassium: 150mg
- Phosphorus: 100mg

Omelet with Spring Onions and Goat's Cheese

Prep Time: 5 minutes | Cook Time: 5 minutes | Serves: 1

Ingredients
- 3 large egg whites
- 1 tablespoon low-fat goat's cheese, crumbled
- 1/4 cup spring onions, finely chopped
- 1 teaspoon olive oil
- Black pepper to taste

Instructions

1. In a bowl, whisk the egg whites until they are frothy and well combined.

2. In a nonstick skillet, warm the olive oil over medium heat. Make sure the pan is evenly coated with oil.

3. Add the finely chopped spring onions to the skillet and sauté for about 2 minutes, until they become soft and fragrant.

4. Pour the whisked egg whites into the skillet, swirling gently to cover the base of the pan.

5. As the eggs begin to set, sprinkle the crumbled goat's cheese evenly over the omelet.

6. Sprinkle a pinch of black pepper over the mixture. Cook until the egg whites are fully set and the cheese is slightly melted, about 2-3 minutes.

7. Carefully fold the omelet in half with a spatula. Serve immediately

Cooking Tips:
- Use low-fat goat's cheese to keep phosphorus levels in check while adding a delightful creaminess to the omelet.
- Ensure you use fresh spring onions and rinse them well to reduce any potential potassium content.

Nutritional Information (per serving):
- Calories: 120
- Protein: 15g
- Carbohydrates: 2g
- Fiber: 0g
- Sodium: 100mg
- Potassium: 150mg
- Phosphorus: 110mg

Burritos Rápidos

Prep Time: 10 minutes | Cook Time: 5 minutes | Serves: 2

Ingredients:
- 2 whole-grain, low-sodium tortillas
- 4 large egg whites
- 1/4 cup diced red bell pepper
- 1/4 cup finely chopped green onions
- 1/4 cup chopped fresh spinach (optional, for added nutrients)
- 2 tablespoons low-fat goat cheese, crumbled
- 1 teaspoon olive oil
- Black pepper to taste

Instructions:
1. In a bowl, whisk the egg whites until they are frothy and well mixed.

2. Warm the olive oil in a non-stick skillet over medium heat, ensuring it coats the pan evenly.

3. Add the diced red bell pepper, green onions, and spinach to the skillet. Sauté for about 2 minutes until they are tender and aromatic.

4. Pour the whisked egg whites into the skillet, stirring gently to combine with the vegetables. Cook until the egg whites are set, approximately 3-4 minutes.

5. Sprinkle the crumbled goat cheese over the cooked eggs and vegetables. Stir gently to mix as the cheese melts slightly.

6. Add a pinch of black pepper to taste. Once the cheese has melted slightly and the eggs are fully cooked, remove the skillet from heat.

7. Place a tortilla on a flat surface. Spoon half of the egg and vegetable mixture onto the center of the tortilla. Fold the sides in and roll up to form a burrito. Repeat with the second tortilla.

Cooking Tips:
- Choose fresh, low-potassium vegetables such as red bell pepper and spinach. Rinse them thoroughly to reduce potassium content further.
- For added flavor, you can sprinkle fresh herbs like cilantro or parsley.
- Make sure to select low-sodium tortillas to keep the sodium content within recommended levels.

Nutritional Information (per serving):
- Calories: 180
- Protein: 10g
- Carbohydrates: 22g
- Fiber: 4g
- Sodium: 150mg
- Potassium: 180mg
- Phosphorus: 120mg

Blueberry Whole Grain Muffins

Prep Time: 15 minutes | Cook Time: 20 minutes | Serves: 12 muffins

Ingredients:
- 1 1/2 cups whole wheat flour
- 1/2 cup rolled oats
- 2 teaspoons low-sodium baking powder
- 1/2 teaspoon baking soda
- 1/4 teaspoon salt
- 1/2 cup unsweetened applesauce
- 1/2 cup unsweetened almond milk
- 1/4 cup olive oil
- 1/2 cup honey or agave syrup
- 1 large egg white
- 1 teaspoon vanilla extract
- 1 cup fresh or frozen blueberries (rinsed and drained if frozen)

Instructions:
1. Set your oven to 375°F (190°C). Line the muffin tin with paper liners or lightly grease it with cooking spray.

2. Mix together the whole wheat flour, rolled oats, low-sodium baking powder, baking soda, and salt in a large mixing bowl.

3. Whisk the unsweetened applesauce, almond milk, olive oil, honey (or agave syrup), egg white, and vanilla extract in a separate bowl until smooth.

4. Pour the wet mixture into the dry mixture and stir gently with a spatula until just combined. If the batter has a few lumps, it's acceptable.

5. Gently fold the blueberries into the batter, ensuring they are evenly dispersed.

6. Divide the batter evenly into the 12 muffin cups, filling each about two-thirds full.

7. Place the muffin tin in the preheated oven and bake for 18-20 minutes, or until a toothpick inserted into the center of a muffin comes out clean.

8. After five minutes of cooling in the muffin tray, move the muffins to a wire rack to finish cooling. Take pleasure in them being heated or room temperature.

Cooking Tips:
- For an added touch, sprinkle some extra rolled oats on top of the muffins before baking.

Nutritional Information
- Calories: 150
- Protein: 3g
- Carbohydrates: 28g
- Fiber: 3g
- Sodium: 80mg
- Potassium: 90mg
- Phosphorus: 60mg

Creamy Garlic Beans on Toast

Prep Time: 10 minutes | Cook Time: 15 minutes | Serves: 2

Ingredients:
- One cup of low-sodium rinsed and drained canned white beans,
- 1/2 cup unsweetened almond milk
- 1 tablespoon olive oil
- 2 cloves garlic, minced
- 1 teaspoon lemon juice
- 1/4 teaspoon dried thyme
- 1/4 teaspoon black pepper
- 2 slices whole-grain, low-sodium bread
- Fresh parsley, chopped (optional, for garnish)

Instructions:

1. Warm up the olive oil in a medium saucepan over medium heat. Add the minced garlic and cook for 1-2 minutes until it becomes fragrant and slightly golden.

2. Add the rinsed and drained white beans to the saucepan. Pour in the unsweetened almond milk and add the lemon juice, dried thyme, and black pepper.

3. Let the bean mixture simmer over medium heat, stirring occasionally, for about 10 minutes. Use a wooden spoon or potato masher to gently mash some of the beans, creating a creamy texture while leaving some whole beans for added texture.

4. While the beans are cooking, toast the slices of whole-grain, low-sodium bread until they are golden and crispy.

5. Once the beans are creamy and heated through, remove the saucepan from heat. Spoon the creamy garlic beans onto the toasted bread slices, dividing evenly between the two servings.

6. Sprinkle with chopped fresh parsley, if desired, for a burst of freshness and color. Serve immediately and enjoy.

Cooking Tips:
- Use low-sodium canned beans and rinse them thoroughly to minimize sodium content.
- For a smoother consistency, you can use an immersion blender to blend the beans slightly before serving.

Nutritional Information (per serving):
- Calories: 220
- Protein: 8g
- Carbohydrates: 34g
- Fiber: 7g
- Sodium: 130mg
- Potassium: 180mg
- Phosphorus: 90mg

Buckwheat Pancakes

Prep Time: 10 minutes | Cook Time: 15 minutes | Serves: 4 (8 pancakes)

Ingredients:
- 1 cup buckwheat flour
- 1/2 cup whole wheat flour
- 2 teaspoons baking powder (low-sodium)
- 1/2 teaspoon baking soda
- 1/4 teaspoon salt
- 1 cup unsweetened almond milk
- 1/4 cup unsweetened applesauce
- 2 tablespoons olive oil
- 1 large egg white
- 1 tablespoon honey or agave syrup
- 1 teaspoon vanilla extract

Instructions:
1. Whisk together the buckwheat flour, whole wheat flour, low-sodium baking powder, baking soda, and salt in a large mixing bowl.

2. Mix together the unsweetened almond milk, unsweetened applesauce, olive oil, egg white, honey (or agave syrup), and vanilla extract in another separate bowl until smooth.

3. Pour the wet ingredients into the dry ingredients and stir gently with a whisk until just combined. Don't overmix; a few lumps are acceptable.

4. Turn up the heat to medium on a nonstick pan or griddle. If needed, very lightly lubricate with a tiny bit of olive oil.

5. For each pancake, pour 1/4 cup of batter onto the griddle. Simmer for two to three minutes, or until surface bubbles appear and the edges seem firm. Cook for a further two to three minutes, or until golden brown on both sides, after flipping.

6. Serve the pancakes warm with your choice of kidney-friendly toppings, such as fresh berries, a drizzle of honey, or a dollop of unsweetened applesauce.

Cooking Tips

- If the batter is too thick, add a little more almond milk to reach your desired consistency.

Nutritional Information (per serving):
- Calories: 140
- Protein: 4g
- Carbohydrates: 26g
- Fiber: 3g
- Sodium: 90mg
- Potassium: 120mg
- Phosphorus: 80mg

Apple Walnut Oatmeal

Prep Time: 5 minutes | Cook Time: 10 minutes | Serves: 2

Ingredients:
- 1 cup rolled oats
- 2 cups unsweetened almond milk
- One medium apple, peeled and diced
- 2 tablespoons chopped walnuts
- 1 tablespoon honey or agave syrup
- 1/2 teaspoon ground cinnamon
- 1/4 teaspoon ground nutmeg
- 1/2 teaspoon vanilla extract

Instructions:

1. In a medium saucepan, bring the unsweetened almond milk to a gentle simmer over medium heat.

2. Stir in the rolled oats and diced apple. Reduce heat to low and cook, stirring occasionally, for about 5-7 minutes, or until the oats are tender and the apples are soft.

3. Stir in the honey (or agave syrup), ground cinnamon, ground nutmeg, and vanilla extract. Cook for an additional 1-2 minutes, until the flavors are well combined and the oatmeal reaches your desired consistency.

4. Remove the saucepan from heat and stir in the chopped walnuts.

Nutritional Information (per serving):
- Calories: 220
- Protein: 6g
- Carbohydrates: 38g
- Fiber: 6g
- Sodium: 20mg
- Potassium: 180mg
- Phosphorus: 90mg

Tropical Fruit Salad with Basil Lime Syrup

Prep Time: 10 minutes | Serves: 2

Ingredients:
- 1 cup pineapple chunks
- 1 cup mango cubes
- 1 cup diced papaya
- 1 cup diced dragon fruit
- 1/2 cup blueberries
- 1/4 cup fresh basil leaves, finely chopped
- 2 tablespoons honey or agave syrup
- 2 tablespoons fresh lime juice
- 1 teaspoon lime zest

Instructions:

1. In a large mixing bowl, combine the pineapple chunks, mango cubes, diced papaya, diced dragon fruit, and blueberries. Toss gently to mix.

2. In a small saucepan, combine the honey (or agave syrup), fresh lime juice, and lime zest. Heat over low heat, stirring occasionally, until the mixture is warmed and the honey is fully dissolved. Remove from heat and stir in the finely chopped basil leaves.

3. Pour the basil lime syrup over the mixed fruits. Gently toss to ensure that the syrup coats every piece of the fruit

4. Let the fruit salad sit for about 10 minutes to allow the flavors to meld together. Serve immediately, or cover and refrigerate for up to 2 hours to enjoy it chilled.

Nutritional Information (per serving):
- Calories: 110
- Protein: 1g
- Carbohydrates: 28g
- Fiber: 3g
- Sodium: 5mg
- Potassium: 150mg
- Phosphorus: 20mg

Tofu Scramble with Veggies

Prep Time: 10 minutes | Cook Time: 10 minutes | Serves: 2

Ingredients:
- 1 block firm tofu, drained and crumbled
- 1 tablespoon olive oil
- 1/2 small red bell pepper, diced
- 1/2 small yellow bell pepper, diced
- 1/2 cup zucchini, diced
- 1/2 small red onion, finely chopped
- 2 cloves garlic, minced
- 1/2 teaspoon ground turmeric
- 1/4 teaspoon ground cumin
- 1/4 teaspoon black pepper
- Fresh parsley, chopped (optional, for garnish)

Instructions:
1. Begin by draining the tofu and crumbling it into small pieces with your hands or a fork. Set aside.

2. Warm up olive oil over medium heat.

3. Add the chopped red bell pepper, yellow bell pepper, zucchini, and red onion to the skillet. The veggies should be sautéed for 3–4 minutes, or until they are soft but still crunchy.

4. Stir in the minced garlic, ground turmeric, ground cumin, and black pepper. Cook until the spices become aromatic, about one more minute.

5. Add the crumbled tofu to the skillet, mixing well with the vegetables and spices. Cook for about 5 minutes, stirring occasionally, until the tofu is heated through and slightly golden.

6. Remove from heat and sprinkle with chopped fresh parsley if desired. Serve hot and enjoy.

Cooking Tips:
- For extra flavor, you can add a splash of low-sodium soy sauce or a squeeze of fresh lemon juice before serving.
- Experiment with other low-potassium vegetables like mushrooms or spinach for variety.

Nutritional Information (per serving):
- Calories: 180
- Protein: 12g
- Carbohydrates: 10g
- Fiber: 3g
- Sodium: 50mg
- Potassium: 220mg
- Phosphorus: 80mg

Baked Peach Oatmeal

Prep Time: 10 minutes | Cook Time: 30 minutes | Serves: 4

Ingredients:
- 2 cups rolled oats

- 1 teaspoon baking powder (low-sodium)
- 1/2 teaspoon ground cinnamon
- 1/4 teaspoon ground nutmeg
- 1 1/2 cups unsweetened almond milk
- 1/4 cup honey or agave syrup
- 1 large egg white
- 1 teaspoon vanilla extract
- 2 medium peaches, diced
- 1/4 cup chopped walnuts (optional)

Instructions:

1. Preheat your oven to 350°F (175°C) and lightly grease an 8x8-inch baking dish.

2. Combine the rolled oats, low-sodium baking powder, ground cinnamon, and ground nutmeg in a mixing bowl.

3. In a separate bowl, whisk together the unsweetened almond milk, honey or agave syrup, egg white, and vanilla extract.

4. Mix the wet and dry ingredients together, stir until it's combined. Gently fold in the diced peaches and optional chopped walnuts.

5. Transfer the mixture into the baking dish that has been preheated and level it out. Bake in the preheated oven for 25-30 minutes, or until the top is golden brown and the oatmeal is set.

6. Allow the baked oatmeal to cool for a few minutes before serving. Cut into squares and enjoy the warmth.

Cooking Tips:

- For an extra touch of sweetness, drizzle a bit of honey or agave syrup on top before serving.
- If fresh peaches are not available, you can use canned peaches; just be sure to choose those packed in juice rather than syrup and rinse them thoroughly.
- This dish can be prepared the night before and baked in the morning for a quick and easy breakfast.

Nutritional Information (per serving):

- Calories: 200

- Protein: 6g
- Carbohydrates: 36g
- Fiber: 5g
- Sodium: 55mg
- Potassium: 150mg
- Phosphorus: 100mg

Lemon Blueberry Corn Muffins

Prep Time: 15 minutes | Cook Time: 20 minutes | Serves: 12

Ingredients:
- 1 cup cornmeal
- 1 cup all-purpose flour
- 1/2 cup granulated sugar
- 1 tablespoon baking powder (low-sodium)
- 1/2 teaspoon baking soda
- 1/4 teaspoon salt
- 1 cup unsweetened almond milk
- 1/4 cup olive oil
- 2 large egg whites
- 1 teaspoon vanilla extract
- 1 tablespoon lemon zest
- 1 cup fresh blueberries

Instructions:
1. Preheat your oven to 375°F (190°C) and line a muffin tin with paper liners.

2. Whisk together the cornmeal, all-purpose flour, granulated sugar, low-sodium baking powder, baking soda, and salt in a large mixing bowl.

3. In a separate bowl, whisk together the unsweetened almond milk, olive oil, egg whites, vanilla extract, and lemon zest until well combined.

4. Mix the wet and dry ingredients together, stir until it's combined. Be careful not to overmix. Gently fold in the fresh blueberries.

5. Spoon the batter evenly into the prepared muffin tin, filling each cup about two-thirds full.

6. When a toothpick is pushed into the center of a muffin, it should come out clean after 18 to 20 minutes of baking in a preheated oven.

7. After letting the muffins cool in the muffin tray for a few minutes, move them to a wire rack to finish cooling. Savor warm or room temperature.

Cooking Tips:
- Frozen blueberries can be substituted for fresh blueberries in this situation. Just remember to thoroughly drain and defrost them before adding them to the batter.
- Leftover muffins can be frozen for extended storage or kept in an airtight container for up to three days.

Nutritional Information (per serving):
- Calories: 150
- Protein: 3g
- Carbohydrates: 25g
- Fiber: 2g
- Sodium: 90mg
- Potassium: 80mg
- Phosphorus: 70mg

Chicken Apple Crunch Salad

Prep Time: 15 minutes | Cook Time: 10 minutes | Serves: 2

Ingredients:
- One large boneless and skinless chicken breast
- 1 tablespoon olive oil
- 1/4 teaspoon black pepper
- 1 teaspoon dried thyme
- One medium apple, thinly sliced
- 1/4 cup chopped celery
- Two cups of mixed greens such as lettuce, arugula, and spinach
- 1/4 cup shredded carrots
- 2 tablespoons chopped walnuts (optional)
- 1/4 cup crumbled goat cheese (optional)
- 2 tablespoons balsamic vinaigrette (low-sodium)

Instructions:
1. In a small bowl, mix the olive oil, black pepper, and dried thyme. Apply the mixture to the chicken breast.

2. A grill pan or skillet should be heated to medium heat. Add the chicken breast and heat until the internal temperature reaches 165°F (75°C), 5 to 6 minutes on each side. Take it from the stove and give it a few minutes to rest before slicing it into thin strips.

3. Combine the mixed greens, sliced apple, chopped celery, and shredded carrots in a mixing bowl.

4. Add the sliced chicken to the salad mixture and combine gently.

5. Sprinkle the chopped walnuts and crumbled goat cheese over the top of the salad if desired.

6. Drizzle the low-sodium balsamic vinaigrette over the salad and stir gently to distribute all ingredients evenly.

Cooking Tips:
- Choose firm, sweet apples like Fuji or Honeycrisp for a crisp texture and sweet flavor.
- For a vegetarian option, substitute the chicken with grilled tofu or chickpeas.
- Adjust the amount of vinaigrette to taste, or make your own using olive oil, balsamic vinegar, and a pinch of herbs.

Nutritional Information (per serving):
- Calories: 250
- Protein: 22g
- Carbohydrates: 18g
- Fiber: 4g
- Sodium: 120mg
- Potassium: 280mg
- Phosphorus: 150mg

Broiled Red Snapper with Herb Pesto

Prep Time: 10 minutes | Cook Time: 15 minutes | Serves: 2

Ingredients:
- 4 oz each of two red snapper filets
- 1 tablespoon olive oil
- 1/4 teaspoon black pepper
- 1/2 lemon, sliced

Herb Pesto:
- 1 cup fresh parsley leaves
- 1/2 cup fresh basil leaves
- 1 clove garlic, minced
- 1/4 cup olive oil
- 2 tablespoons lemon juice
- 1 tablespoon pine nuts or walnuts
- 1/4 teaspoon black pepper

Instructions:
1. Preheat your broiler to high and line a baking sheet with aluminum foil.

2. Pat the red snapper filets dry with paper towels. Brush both sides with olive oil and season with black pepper.

3. When the fish is opaque and flakes readily with a fork, place the filets on the prepared baking sheet and broil for 6 to 8 minutes on each side.

4. While the fish is broiling, prepare the herb pesto. In a food processor or blender, combine the parsley, basil, minced garlic, olive oil, lemon juice, pine nuts or walnuts, and black pepper. Blend until smooth.

5. Transfer the broiled red snapper filets to plates. Spoon the herb pesto over the top of each filet. Garnish with lemon slices.

6. Serve with a side of steamed vegetables or a light salad.

Cooking Tips:
- For a nut-free version, omit the nuts from the pesto and add a bit more herbs for texture.
- Pair this dish with a simple side like steamed green beans or a mixed greens salad for a complete meal.

Nutritional Information (per serving):
- Calories: 320
- Protein: 25g
- Carbohydrates: 4g
- Fiber: 1g
- Sodium: 60mg
- Potassium: 400mg
- Phosphorus: 200mg

Apple Rice Salad

Prep Time: 15mins | Cook Time: 20 mins | Serves: 4

Ingredients:
- 1 cup uncooked white rice
- 2 medium apples, diced
- 1/2 cup diced celery
- 1/4 cup chopped fresh parsley
- 1/4 cup chopped walnuts (optional)
- 2 tablespoons dried cranberries
- 3 tablespoons olive oil
- 2 tablespoons apple cider vinegar
- 1 tablespoon honey
- 1 teaspoon Dijon mustard (low-sodium)
- 1/4 teaspoon black pepper

Instructions

1. Two cups of water should be brought to a boil in a medium saucepan. When the rice is soft and the water has been absorbed, add the rice, lower the heat to low, cover, and simmer for about 18 to 20 minutes. Take it off the stove and let it come to room temperature.

2. Mix together the olive oil, apple cider vinegar, honey, Dijon mustard, and black pepper in a bowl until well combined.

3. In another bowl, combine the cooked rice, diced apples, diced celery, chopped parsley, chopped walnuts (if using), and dried cranberries.

4. After adding the dressing to the rice mixture, carefully toss to coat all of the ingredients.

5. Transfer the salad to a serving bowl and serve immediately, or chill in the refrigerator for about 30 minutes to allow the flavors to meld.

Cooking Tips:
- For extra flavor, you can toast the walnuts in a dry skillet over medium heat for a few minutes before adding them to the salad.

- This salad can be made ahead of time and stored in the refrigerator for up to 2 days.

Nutritional Information (per serving):
- Calories: 250
- Protein: 4g
- Carbohydrates: 40g
- Fiber: 3g
- Sodium: 20mg
- Potassium: 150mg
- Phosphorus: 90mg

Pumpkin and Carrot Soup

Prep Time: 15mins | Cook Time: 30 mins | Serves: 4

Ingredients:
- 2 cups pumpkin, peeled and diced
- 2 cups carrots, peeled and sliced
- 1 small onion, chopped
- 2 cloves garlic, minced
- 1 tablespoon olive oil
- Four cups low-sodium vegetable broth
- 1 teaspoon dried thyme
- 1/4 teaspoon black pepper
- 1/4 cup unsweetened almond milk (optional, for creaminess)
- Fresh parsley, chopped (for garnish)

Instructions:
1. Peel and dice the pumpkin and carrots. Finely chop the onion and the garlic.

2. Heat the olive oil in a big pot over medium heat. Add the chopped onion and minced garlic, and sauté for 3–4 minutes, or until the onion is transparent and fragrant.

3. Include the sliced carrots and diced pumpkin in the pot. Stir in the black pepper and dried thyme, then pour in the low-sodium vegetable broth. Mix thoroughly to blend.

4. After bringing the mixture to a boil, turn down the heat. When the vegetables are soft, around 20 to 25 minutes of simmering time is recommended.

5. Blend the soup with an immersion blender until it's creamy and smooth. In case you lack an immersion blender, you may move the soup into a blender in small portions and process it until it becomes smooth, then put it back into the pot.

6. Stir in the unsweetened almond milk for added creaminess. Heat through for another 2-3 minutes, but do not boil.

Cooking Tips:
- You can use canned pumpkin puree if fresh pumpkin is not available; just be sure it's pure pumpkin without added sugars or spices.
- Adjust the consistency of the soup by adding more or less broth according to your preference.
- For added flavor, you can roast the pumpkin and carrots before adding them to the soup.

Nutritional Information (per serving):
- Calories: 120
- Protein: 2g
- Carbohydrates: 20g
- Fiber: 4g
- Sodium: 50mg
- Potassium: 300mg
- Phosphorus: 60mg

Broccoli Chicken Casserole

Prep Time: 15 minutes | Cook Time: 35 minutes | Serves: 6

Ingredients:
- Two cups cooked chicken breast, shredded
- 4 cups broccoli florets
- One cup of low-sodium chicken broth
- 1 cup unsweetened almond milk

- 1/4 cup plain Greek yogurt
- 2 cloves garlic, minced
- 1/2 teaspoon onion powder
- 1/2 teaspoon dried thyme
- 1/4 teaspoon black pepper
- 1 cup shredded low-fat cheddar cheese
- 1/4 cup grated Parmesan cheese
- 2 cups cooked brown rice

Instructions:

1. Preheat your oven to 375°F (190°C). Apply cooking spray to the casserole dish.

2. In a large skillet, steam the broccoli florets with a splash of water over medium heat for about 3-4 minutes, until tender-crisp. Remove excess water and place aside

3. Whisk together the low-sodium chicken broth, unsweetened almond milk, plain Greek yogurt, minced garlic, onion powder, dried thyme, and black pepper in a mixing bowl until smooth.

4. In the greased casserole dish, layer the cooked chicken breast, steamed broccoli florets, and cooked brown rice. Pour the sauce mixture evenly over the top.

5. Sprinkle the shredded low-fat cheddar cheese and grated Parmesan cheese over the casserole.

6. Cover the casserole dish with foil and bake in the preheated oven for 25 minutes. After that, take off the foil and bake for a further ten minutes, or until the cheese is bubbling and melted.

7. Before serving, let the casserole cool for a few minutes. Serve hot and enjoy!

Cooking Tips:
- For convenience, you may use rotisserie chicken or leftover cooked chicken.
- Feel free to substitute other low-potassium vegetables like cauliflower or green beans for the broccoli.
- For a gluten-free option, use quinoa or gluten-free pasta instead of brown rice.

Nutritional Information (per serving):
- Calories: 250

- Protein: 25g
- Carbohydrates: 20g
- Fiber: 3g
- Sodium: 200mg
- Potassium: 300mg
- Phosphorus: 200mg

Lemon Curry Chicken Salad

Prep Time: 20 minutes | Cook Time: 10 minutes | Serves: 4

Ingredients:
- 2 cups cooked chicken breast, diced
- 1/2 cup plain Greek yogurt
- 2 tablespoons mayonnaise (low-sodium)
- 1 tablespoon fresh lemon juice
- 1 teaspoon lemon zest
- 1 teaspoon curry powder
- 1/4 teaspoon black pepper
- 1/4 cup diced celery
- 1/4 cup diced red bell pepper
- 2 tablespoons chopped fresh parsley
- 2 tablespoons unsweetened dried cranberries

Instructions:

1. If not using leftover chicken, cook the chicken breast by boiling or baking until fully cooked. Allow to cool, then dice into small cubes.

2. Combine the plain Greek yogurt, low-sodium mayonnaise, fresh lemon juice, lemon zest, curry powder, and black pepper. Whisk until smooth and well combined.

3. Add the diced chicken, diced celery, diced red bell pepper, chopped parsley, and unsweetened dried cranberries to the bowl with the dressing. After adding the dressing, carefully toss to coat all of the ingredients

4. To let the flavors mingle, cover the bowl and chill it in the refrigerator for at least thirty minutes. Serve the salad chilled.

Serving Suggestions:
- Serve it in a whole grain wrap or pita for a delicious sandwich option.
- Pair with a side of sliced cucumbers or bell pepper strips for added crunch.

Nutritional Information (per serving):
- Calories: 180
- Protein: 20g
- Carbohydrates: 10g
- Fiber: 2g
- Sodium: 150mg
- Potassium: 220mg
- Phosphorus: 180mg

BBQ Lemon and Dill Salmon

Prep Time: 10 minutes | Cook Time: 15 minutes | Serves: 4

Ingredients:
- 4 salmon filets about 4-6 oz each
- 2 tablespoons olive oil
- 2 tablespoons fresh lemon juice
- 2 cloves garlic, minced
- 1 tablespoon chopped fresh dill
- 1/2 teaspoon paprika
- 1/4 teaspoon black pepper
- 2 tablespoons low-sodium barbecue sauce

Instructions:
1. Warm up your grill or grill pan to medium-high heat.

2. Utilizing paper towels, pat the salmon filets dry. To make marinade, combine olive oil, fresh lemon juice, minced garlic, chopped fresh dill, paprika, and black pepper in a mixing bowl.

3. After the salmon filets are thoroughly coated, place them in the marinade. Allow them to marinate for approximately ten minutes at room temperature, or up to thirty minutes in the refrigerator for a stronger flavor.

4. To avoid sticking, lightly oil the grill grates after it has heated up. Skin-side down, put the salmon filets on the grill. The salmon should be cooked through and flake easily with a fork after 4–5 minutes of cooking on each side.

5. During the last few minutes of cooking, brush the top of each salmon filet with a thin layer of low-sodium barbecue sauce. Allow the sauce to caramelize slightly on the salmon.

Serving Suggestions:
- Pair the BBQ Lemon and Dill Salmon with a side of steamed vegetables or a crisp green salad for a balanced meal.
- Serve with a whole grain pilaf or quinoa for added fiber and nutrients.
- Enjoy leftovers cold over a bed of mixed greens for a refreshing salmon salad.

Cooking Tips:
- Ensure the grill is well-heated before adding the salmon to achieve beautiful grill marks and prevent sticking.
- Use a basting brush to apply the barbecue sauce evenly and avoid flare-ups on the grill.

Nutritional Information (per serving):
- Calories: 250
- Protein: 25g
- Carbohydrates: 2g
- Fiber: 0g
- Sodium: 100mg
- Potassium: 400mg
- Phosphorus: 250mg

Chicken Broth

Prep Time: 10 minutes | Cook Time: 2-3 hours | Makes: Approximately 8 cups

Ingredients:
- 1 whole chicken (about 3-4 lbs), preferably organic
- 1 onion, peeled and quartered
- 2 carrots, washed and chopped
- 2 celery stalks, washed and chopped
- 4 cloves garlic, smashed
- 1 bay leaf
- 1 teaspoon whole peppercorns
- Water, enough to cover the ingredients

Instructions:

1. Rinse the whole chicken under cold water and remove any excess fat or giblets from the cavity. Put the chicken in a stock pot.

2. Add the quartered onion, chopped carrots, chopped celery, smashed garlic cloves, bay leaf, and whole peppercorns to the stockpot with the chicken.

3. Pour enough water into the stockpot to cover all the ingredients by about 2 inches. The exact amount will vary depending on the size of your pot and chicken.

4. Place the stockpot over medium heat and slowly bring the mixture to a gentle simmer. Using a spoon, skim off any froth or particles that come to the top.

5. Once the broth reaches a simmer, reduce the heat to low and cover the pot partially with a lid. Let the broth simmer gently for 2-3 hours, stirring occasionally.

6. After simmering, carefully remove the chicken and vegetables from the broth using a slotted spoon or tongs. Discard the solids. If desired, strain the broth through a cheesecloth or fine mesh strainer to remove any remaining particles.

7. Allow the broth to cool slightly before transferring it to storage containers. Refrigerate the broth for up to 4-5 days, or freeze it for longer storage.

Serving Suggestions:
- Enjoy the Homemade Chicken Broth as a comforting and nourishing drink on its own.
- Use it as a base for soups, stews, sauces, or gravies to enhance their flavor and nutritional value.

- Substitute it for water in recipes like rice, quinoa, or couscous for added depth of flavor.

Cooking Tips:
- For a richer broth, roast the chicken and vegetables in the oven before adding them to the stockpot.
- Customize the broth by adding herbs like parsley, thyme, or rosemary for additional flavor.

Nutritional Information (per cup):
- Calories: 15
- Protein: 2g
- Carbohydrates: 1g
- Fat: 1g
- Sodium: 50mg
- Potassium: 40mg
- Phosphorus: 15mg

Mushroom Broth

Prep Time: 10 minutes | Cook Time: 1-2 hours | Makes: Approximately 6 cups

Ingredients:
- 1 lb assorted mushrooms (such as button, cremini, or shiitake), cleaned and sliced
- 1 onion, peeled and quartered
- 2 carrots, washed and chopped
- 2 celery stalks, washed and chopped
- 4 cloves garlic, smashed
- 1 bay leaf
- 1 teaspoon whole peppercorns
- Water, enough to cover the ingredients

Instructions
1. Clean the mushrooms with a damp cloth or brush to remove any dirt. Slice the mushrooms into even pieces after trimming the stems.

2.   In a large stockpot, combine the sliced mushrooms, quartered onion, chopped carrots, chopped celery, smashed garlic cloves, bay leaf, and whole peppercorns.

3. Pour enough water into the stockpot to cover all the ingredients by about 2 inches. The exact amount will vary depending on the size of your pot and mushrooms.

4.   Place the stockpot over medium heat and slowly bring the mixture to a gentle simmer. Using a spoon, skim off any froth or particles that come to the top.

5. Once the broth reaches a simmer, reduce the heat to low and cover the pot partially with a lid. Let the broth simmer gently for 1-2 hours, stirring occasionally.

6. After simmering, carefully remove the solids from the broth using a slotted spoon or tongs. If desired, strain the broth through a cheesecloth or fine mesh strainer to remove any remaining particles.

7. Allow the broth to cool slightly before transferring it to storage containers. Refrigerate the broth for up to 4-5 days, or freeze it for longer storage.

Serving Suggestions:
- Enjoy the Homemade Mushroom Broth as a flavorful and comforting drink on its own.
- Use it as a base for mushroom soup, risotto, or gravy to enhance their savory notes.
- Add depth of flavor to sauces, marinades, or braises by incorporating this rich mushroom broth.

Nutritional Information (per cup):
- Calories: 15
- Protein: 1g
- Carbohydrates: 3g
- Fiber: 1g
- Fat: 0g
- Sodium: 10mg
- Potassium: 100mg
- Phosphorus: 20mg

Honey Molasses Pork

Prep Time: 10 minutes | Cook Time: 30 minutes | Serves: 4

Ingredients:
- One lb pork tenderloin, trimmed of excess fat
- 2 tablespoons honey
- 1 tablespoon molasses
- 2 cloves garlic, minced
- One tablespoon low-sodium soy sauce
- 1 teaspoon grated fresh ginger
- 1/2 teaspoon black pepper
- 1 tablespoon olive oil
- Fresh parsley, chopped (for garnish)

Instructions:

1. Slice the pork tenderloin into 1-inch thick medallions. Add black pepper to the pork on both sides

2. Combine the honey, molasses, minced garlic, low-sodium soy sauce, and grated fresh ginger in a bowl. Whisk until well combined.

3. Place the pork medallions in the marinade, ensuring they are evenly coated. Let them marinate for at least 10 minutes at room temperature, or refrigerate for up to 1 hour for a deeper flavor.

4. Warm up the olive oil in a skillet or grill pan over medium-high heat. Add the marinated pork medallions to the skillet and cook for about 3-4 minutes on each side, or until golden brown and cooked through. Make sure the pork achieves an internal temperature of 145°F, or 63°C.

5. During the last few minutes of cooking, use a basting brush to glaze the pork medallions with the remaining marinade. Let them cook for another minute on each side to caramelize the glaze slightly.

Serving Suggestions:

- Serve the Honey Molasses Pork with steamed vegetables and brown rice for a balanced meal.
- Pair it with a side salad dressed with a light vinaigrette for a refreshing accompaniment.
- Enjoy leftovers cold sliced thinly in sandwiches or wraps for a quick and tasty lunch option.

Cooking Tips:
- Be careful not to overcook the pork tenderloin to ensure it remains tender and juicy.
- If grilling outdoors, preheat the grill to medium-high heat and grill the pork medallions for 3-4 minutes on each side, basting with the marinade as directed.
- Adjust the sweetness of the dish by varying the amount of honey and molasses according to your taste preferences.

Nutritional Information (per serving):
- Calories: 200
- Protein: 25g
- Carbohydrates: 10g
- Fiber: 0g
- Fat: 6g
- Sodium: 100mg
- Potassium: 350mg
- Phosphorus: 200mg

Tuna Macaroni Salad

Prep Time: 15 minutes | Cook Time: 10 minutes | Serves: 4

Ingredients:
- Two cups of uncooked elbow macaroni pasta
- Two cans of 5 oz each tuna in water, drained
- 1/2 cup diced celery
- 1/2 cup of red bell pepper, diced
- 1/4 cup diced red onion
- 1/4 cup chopped fresh parsley
- 1/2 cup plain Greek yogurt
- Two tablespoons of low sodium mayonnaise

- 1 tablespoon lemon juice
- 1 teaspoon Dijon mustard (low-sodium)
- 1/4 teaspoon black pepper
- Salt to taste

Instructions:

1. Cook the elbow macaroni pasta as directed on the package, or until al dente, in a large pot of boiling salted water. Drain the pasta in a sieve and rinse with cold water to halt the cooking process. Let the spaghetti cool completely.

2. Incorporate the plain Greek yogurt, lemon juice, Dijon mustard, low-sodium mayonnaise, black pepper, and salt according to taste. Blend the dressing until it's well-combined and smooth.

3. Add the cooked and cooled elbow macaroni pasta, drained tuna, diced celery, diced red bell pepper, diced red onion, and chopped fresh parsley in a large mixing bowl.

4. Transfer the ready-made dressing to the mixing bowl with the salad ingredients. Toss gently until all the ingredients are equally coated with the dressing, using a mixing spoon.

5. Cover the bowl with plastic wrap and refrigerate the tuna macaroni salad for at least 30 minutes to allow the flavors to meld together. Serve chilled and enjoy!

Cooking Tips:

- For a creamier dressing, adjust the ratio of Greek yogurt to mayonnaise according to your preference.
- Customize the salad by adding other vegetables such as diced cucumbers, shredded carrots, or halved cherry tomatoes.
- Make sure to drain the tuna well to remove excess water and prevent the salad from becoming too watery.

Nutritional Information (per serving):

- Calories: 250
- Protein: 20g
- Carbohydrates: 30g
- Fiber: 3g
- Fat: 5g

- Sodium: 200mg
- Potassium: 250mg
- Phosphorus: 200mg

Turkey Burger

Prep Time: 10 minutes | Cook Time: 15 minutes | Serves: 4

Ingredients:
- One lb lean ground turkey
- 1/4 cup finely chopped onion
- 2 cloves garlic, minced
- 1 tablespoon chopped fresh parsley
- 1 teaspoon dried oregano
- 1/2 teaspoon paprika
- 1/2 teaspoon black pepper
- 1/4 teaspoon salt (optional)
- 4 whole grain burger buns
- Lettuce leaves and onion slices for garnish

Instructions:

1. In a mixing bowl, combine the lean ground turkey, finely chopped onion, minced garlic, chopped fresh parsley, dried oregano, paprika, black pepper, and salt (if using). Use your hands to mix until all the ingredients are evenly incorporated.

2. Divide the turkey mixture into 4 equal portions. Shape each portion into a round patty, about 1/2-inch thick. Press gently in the center to create an indentation, which will prevent the burgers from puffing up during cooking.

3. Preheat a grill or skillet over medium heat. Place the turkey burger patties on the grill or skillet and cook for about 6-7 minutes on each side, or until they are cooked through and no longer pink in the center. Use a spatula to flip the burgers halfway through cooking.

4. Toast the whole grain burger buns lightly, if desired. Top each bread with a turkey burger patty on the bottom half. Add pieces of onion, and lettuce on top. Place the top half of the bun on top.

5. Serve the turkey burgers immediately, accompanied by your favorite side dishes such as sweet potato fries, coleslaw, or a mixed green salad.

Serving Suggestions:
- Customize your turkey burger by adding toppings such as avocado slices, roasted red peppers, or grilled mushrooms.
- Serve with condiments like mustard, ketchup, or a homemade yogurt-based sauce for extra flavor.
- Enjoy the turkey burgers wrapped in lettuce leaves for a low-carb option.

Cooking Tips:
- Make sure the turkey burger patties are cooked to an internal temperature of 165°F (75°C) for safe consumption.
- Avoid pressing down on the burger patties with a spatula while cooking, as this can cause them to lose their juices and become dry.
- For extra flavor, marinate the turkey burger patties in your favorite herbs and spices for 30 minutes before cooking.

Nutritional Information (per serving, without bun and toppings):
- Calories: 150
- Protein: 20g
- Carbohydrates: 2g
- Fat: 7g
- Sodium: 80mg
- Potassium: 200mg
- Phosphorus: 150mg

Lamb and Barley Casserole

Prep Time: 20 minutes | Cook Time: 2 hours | Serves: 6

Ingredients:
- One lb lamb stew meat, diced
- 1 cup pearl barley, rinsed
- 1 onion, diced
- 2 carrots, peeled and diced
- 2 celery stalks, diced

- 2 cloves garlic, minced
- 1 teaspoon dried thyme
- 1 teaspoon dried rosemary
- Four cups of low-sodium beef or vegetable broth
- Salt and black pepper to taste
- Chopped fresh parsley for garnish

Instructions:

1. Heat a large Dutch oven or oven-safe pot over medium-high heat. Add the diced lamb stew meat to the pot and cook, stirring occasionally, until browned on all sides, about 5-7 minutes. Remove the browned lamb from the pot and set aside.

2. Add the diced onion, carrots, celery, and minced garlic inside the same pot. Cook, stirring occasionally, until the vegetables are softened, for about 5 minutes.

3. Return the browned lamb to the pot with the sauteed vegetables. Add the rinsed pearl barley, dried thyme, and dried rosemary to the pot. Season with salt and black pepper to taste.

4. Into the pot with the ingredients thoroughly submerged, pour the low-sodium beef or vegetable broth. Once you have brought the mixture to a boil, turn down the heat to low and place a lid on the pot. Simmer, stirring from time to time, until the barley is cooked through and the lamb is tender, about 1 1/2 to 2 hours.

5. Once the lamb and barley are cooked to perfection, remove the pot from the heat. Taste and adjust the seasoning if necessary. Serve the casserole hot, garnished with chopped fresh parsley for a burst of color and flavor.

Serving Suggestions:

- Enjoy the Lamb and Barley Casserole as a complete meal on its own, or pair it with a side salad or steamed vegetables for added freshness.
- Serve the casserole with a slice of crusty whole grain bread for a hearty and satisfying lunch.
- Freeze leftovers in individual portions for convenient meals later on.

Cooking Tips:

- For added flavor, sear the lamb in batches to ensure even browning and caramelization.
- Use low-sodium broth to control the sodium content of the dish and support kidney health.

Nutritional Information (per serving):
- Calories: 300
- Protein: 20g
- Carbohydrates: 30g
- Fiber: 6g
- Fat: 10g
- Sodium: 150mg
- Potassium: 350mg
- Phosphorus: 200mg

Creamy Cauliflower and Pear Soup

Prep Time: 10 mins | Cook Time: 25 mins | Serves: 4

Ingredients:
- One head cauliflower, chopped
- 2 ripe pears, chopped
- 1 onion, diced
- 2 cloves garlic, minced
- Four cups of low-sodium vegetable broth
- 1/2 teaspoon ground nutmeg
- Salt and black pepper to taste
- 2 tablespoons olive oil
- Fresh parsley for garnish

Instructions:
1. Warm up the olive oil in a big pot over medium heat. Cook for three to four minutes, or until the ingredients are tender and aromatic, after adding the chopped onion and minced garlic.

2. Include chopped pears and cauliflower florets in the pot. Cook for a further five minutes, stirring occasionally, or until the cauliflower begins to soften.

3. Add the low-sodium vegetable broth and adjust the seasoning to taste with salt, black pepper, and ground nutmeg. Once the cauliflower and pears are soft, reduce the heat to a simmer and cook for 15 to 20 minutes.

4. After the pears and cauliflower are cooked through, purée the soup until it's creamy and smooth using a blender or immersion blender. When combining hot liquids, exercise caution.

5. You can adjust the soup's consistency by adding extra water or vegetable broth if it's too thick. You can boil it for a few more minutes to thicken it if it's too thin.

6. If preferred, garnish with finely chopped fresh parsley or chives. Enjoy it while it's hot!

Serving Suggestions:
- Serve the Creamy Cauliflower and Pear Soup with crusty whole grain bread or garlic croutons for added texture and flavor.
- Pair with a crisp green salad dressed with a light vinaigrette for a refreshing contrast.
- Drizzle with a swirl of plain Greek yogurt or a dollop of low-fat sour cream for extra creaminess.

Cooking Tips:
- Choose ripe pears for a sweeter flavor profile in the soup. If your pears are not fully ripe, you can add a touch of honey or maple syrup to enhance the sweetness.
- For an extra flavor, roast the cauliflower florets and pears in the oven before adding them to the soup.
- Store any leftover soup in an airtight container in the refrigerator for up to 3 days. Reheat gently on the stovetop or in the microwave before serving.

Nutritional Information (per serving):
- Calories: 150
- Protein: 4g
- Carbohydrates: 20g
- Fiber: 5g
- Fat: 7g
- Sodium: 200mg
- Potassium: 400mg
- Phosphorus: 100mg

DINNER RECIPES

Zucchini Carrot Soup

Prep Time: 10 minutes | Cook Time: 25 minutes | Serves: 4

Ingredients:
- 2 tablespoons olive oil
- 1 onion, chopped
- 3 cloves garlic, minced
- 4 large carrots, peeled and sliced
- 2 medium zucchinis, chopped
- Four cups of low-sodium vegetable broth
- 1 teaspoon dried thyme
- 1 teaspoon dried oregano
- Salt and black pepper to taste
- Fresh parsley for garnish

Instructions:
1. Warm up the olive oil in a big pot over medium heat. Cook for three to four minutes, or until the ingredients are tender and aromatic, after adding the chopped onion and minced garlic.

2. Stir in the sliced carrots and chopped zucchini, cooking for another 5 minutes until they begin to soften.

3. Add the low-sodium vegetable broth and adjust the seasoning to taste with dried thyme, and dried oregano. Once the vegetables are soft, reduce the heat to a simmer and cook for 15 to 20 minutes.,

4. Once the vegetables are cooked, Blend the soup with an immersion blender until it's creamy and smooth. Be careful when blending hot liquids.

5. Season the soup with salt and black pepper to taste. Adjust the seasoning as needed.

6. Serve the zucchini carrot soup into bowls and garnish with fresh parsley. Serve hot and enjoy!

Serving Suggestions:
- Pair the Zucchini Carrot Soup with a slice of whole grain bread or a small side salad for a complete meal.
- Add a dollop of plain Greek yogurt or a sprinkle of low-fat feta cheese for added creaminess and flavor.
- Serve with a light, refreshing cucumber and tomato salad dressed with lemon juice and olive oil.

Nutritional Information (per serving):
- Calories: 130
- Protein: 3g
- Carbohydrates: 17g
- Fiber: 4g
- Fat: 7g
- Sodium: 150mg
- Potassium: 500mg
- Phosphorus: 50mg

Chicken Stew with Mushroom and Kale

Prep Time: 15 minutes | Cook Time: 40 minutes | Serves: 4

Ingredients:
- One lb boneless and skinless chicken thighs, cut into bite-sized pieces
- 2 tablespoons olive oil
- 1 onion, diced
- 3 cloves garlic, minced
- 8 oz mushrooms, sliced
- One bunch of kale, chopped
- Four cups of low-sodium chicken broth
- 2 carrots, sliced

- 2 stalks celery, sliced
- 1 teaspoon dried thyme
- 1 teaspoon dried rosemary
- 1/2 teaspoon ground black pepper
- Fresh parsley for garnish (optional)

Instructions:

1. Warm up the olive oil in a big pot or dutch oven over medium heat. Cook for three to four minutes, or until the ingredients are tender and aromatic, after adding the chopped onion and minced garlic.

2. Add the chicken pieces to the pot, cooking until browned on all sides, about 5-7 minutes.

3. Stir in the sliced mushrooms, carrots, and celery. Cook until the veggies start to soften, about 5 more minutes.

4. Add the low-sodium vegetable broth and adjust the seasoning to taste with dried thyme, dried rosemary and ground black pepper. Bring the mixture to a simmer.

5. Once the stew reaches a simmer, reduce the heat to low and cover the pot partially with a lid. Let the stew simmer gently for 20 minutes, stirring occasionally

6. Stir in the chopped kale, and continue to simmer for another 5 minutes until the kale is wilted and tender.

7. Put the chicken stew into bowls. If desired, garnish with fresh parsley. Serve hot and enjoy!

Serving Suggestions:
- Serve the Chicken Stew with a side of whole grain bread or a slice of crusty baguette for dipping.
- Pair with a light green salad dressed with a simple vinaigrette for a balanced meal.

Nutritional Information (per serving):
- Calories: 280
- Protein: 30g
- Carbohydrates: 12g
- Fiber: 4g

- Fat: 12g
- Sodium: 200mg
- Potassium: 500mg
- Phosphorus: 250mg

Grilled Lemon Chicken Kebabs

Prep Time: 15 minutes (plus marinating time) | Cook Time: 15 minutes | Serves: 4

Ingredients:
- One lb boneless and skinless chicken breasts, cut into bite-sized pieces
- 1/4 cup olive oil
- 1/4 cup fresh lemon juice
- 2 tablespoons chopped fresh parsley
- 1 tablespoon chopped fresh rosemary
- 2 cloves garlic, minced
- 1 teaspoon lemon zest
- 1/2 teaspoon ground black pepper
- Wooden skewers (soaked in water for 30 minutes)

Instructions:
1. Combine olive oil, fresh lemon juice, chopped parsley, chopped rosemary, minced garlic, lemon zest, and ground black pepper in a mixing bowl. Whisk until well blended.

2. Add the chicken pieces to the bowl with the marinade, stirring to coat evenly. If you want a stronger flavor, cover and chill for up to two hours, but at least thirty minutes is preferred.

3. A grill pan or skillet should be heated to medium heat.

4. Thread the marinated chicken pieces onto the soaked wooden skewers, leaving a little space between each piece to ensure even cooking.

5. Place the kebabs on the preheated grill. Cook for about 10-15 minutes, turning occasionally, until the chicken is cooked through and has nice grill marks.

6. Remove the kebabs from the grill and let rest for a few minutes. Serve hot, If desired, garnish with additional chopped fresh parsley and lemon wedges

Serving Suggestions:
- Pair the Grilled Lemon Chicken Kebabs with a side of steamed green beans or a mixed green salad for a balanced meal.
- Serve with a side of quinoa or brown rice for added fiber and nutrition.
- For a Mediterranean twist, serve with a dollop of tzatziki sauce and a side of grilled vegetables.

Cooking Tips:
- For extra flavor, you can add vegetables such as bell peppers, cherry tomatoes, and zucchini to the skewers.
- If you don't have fresh herbs on hand, you can use dried herbs, but reduce the quantity by half as they are more concentrated.
- Make sure to soak the wooden skewers in water to prevent them from burning on the grill.

Nutritional Information (per serving):
- Calories: 250
- Protein: 28g
- Carbohydrates: 3g
- Fiber: 0g
- Fat: 14g
- Sodium: 80mg
- Potassium: 400mg
- Phosphorus: 220mg

Baked Tilapia Fillet with Gremolata

Prep Time: 10 minutes | Cook Time: 20 minutes | Serves: 4

Ingredients:
- 4 tilapia filets
- 2 tablespoons olive oil
- Salt and black pepper to taste
- 1 cup fresh parsley, finely chopped

- 2 cloves garlic, minced
- Zest of 1 lemon
- 1 tablespoon lemon juice

Instructions:
1. Preheat the oven to 375°F (190°C).

2. Grease the baking dish with 1 tablespoon of olive oil. Place the tilapia filets in the dish, and season with a small amount of salt and black pepper.

3. The salmon should be cooked through and flake easily with a fork after 15-20 minutes of cooking on each side.

4. While the fish is baking, prepare the gremolata. Mix the chopped parsley, minced garlic, lemon zest, and lemon juice in a bowl. Add the final tablespoon of olive oil and stir.

5. Once the tilapia is cooked, remove it from the oven and spoon the gremolata evenly over each filet.

6. Garnish with fresh parsley and serve.

Serving Suggestions:
- Pair the Baked Tilapia Fillet with Gremolata with a side of steamed green beans or roasted asparagus for a balanced meal.
- Serve with a simple quinoa or brown rice pilaf for added fiber and nutrients.
- Complement the dish with a mixed greens salad dressed with a light lemon vinaigrette.

Nutritional Information (per serving):
- Calories: 200
- Protein: 23g
- Carbohydrates: 2g
- Fiber: 1g
- Fat: 11g
- Sodium: 120mg
- Potassium: 450mg
- Phosphorus: 200mg

Couscous Salad with Roasted Vegetables

Prep Time: 15 minutes | Cook Time: 30 minutes | Serves: 4

Ingredients:
- 1 cup whole wheat couscous
- One 1/4 cups low-sodium vegetable broth
- 1 zucchini, chopped
- 1 red bell pepper, chopped
- 1 yellow bell pepper, chopped
- 1 red onion, chopped
- 1 cup cherry tomatoes, halved
- 2 tablespoons olive oil
- 1 teaspoon dried oregano
- 1 teaspoon dried basil
- Black pepper to taste
- Juice of 1 lemon
- 1/4 cup fresh parsley, chopped

Instructions:
1. Preheat the oven to 400°F (200°C).

2. Arrange the diced zucchini, cherry tomatoes, red and yellow bell peppers, and red onion on a baking sheet. Add a drizzle of 1 tablespoon olive oil and season with black pepper, dried basil, and dried oregano. For an even coat, toss.

3. Roast the veggies, stirring halfway through, in the preheated oven for 25 to 30 minutes, or until they are soft and beginning to caramelize.

4. In a medium saucepan, bring the low-sodium vegetable broth to a boil while the veggies roast. Remove from heat, cover, and stir in the couscous. Use a fork to fluff it after five minutes.

5. Mix the cooked couscous with the roasted vegetables in a bowl. Add the remaining 1 tablespoon of olive oil, lemon juice, and chopped parsley. Toss gently to combine. Serve

Serving Suggestions:
- Pair the Couscous Salad with a side of grilled chicken or fish for added protein.
- Serve alongside a simple cucumber and yogurt salad for a refreshing contrast.

Cooking Tips:
- If you prefer a bit of sweetness, add a handful of dried cranberries or raisins to the salad.

Nutritional Information (per serving):
- Calories: 220
- Protein: 6g
- Carbohydrates: 34g
- Fiber: 6g
- Fat: 8g
- Sodium: 80mg
- Potassium: 450mg
- Phosphorus: 100mg

Fish Tacos

Prep Time: 20 minutes | Cook Time: 10 minutes | Serves: 4

Ingredients:
- One lb white fish filets (such as tilapia or cod)
- 2 tablespoons olive oil
- 1 teaspoon ground cumin
- 1 teaspoon paprika
- 1/2 teaspoon ground black pepper
- 8 small corn tortillas
- 2 cups shredded green cabbage
- 1 cup shredded carrots
- 1/4 cup fresh cilantro, chopped
- Juice of 2 limes
- 1 tablespoon apple cider vinegar
- 1 tablespoon honey
- 1 avocado, sliced (optional)

- Lime wedges for serving

Instructions
1. Pat the fish filets dry with paper towels. In a small bowl, mix together the ground cumin, paprika, and black pepper. Rub the seasoning mixture evenly over both sides of the fish filets.

2. A big pan filled with one tablespoon of olive oil is heated to medium-high heat. When the fish is opaque and flakes easily with a fork, add the filets and fry for about 3–4 minutes on each side. Take out and place aside from the skillet.

3. Combine the chopped cilantro, shredded carrots, and shredded green cabbage in a mixing dish. Whisk together the remaining tablespoon of olive oil, honey, apple cider vinegar, and the juice from one lime in a separate small bowl. Drizzle the cabbage mixture with the dressing, then toss to coat.

4. In the same skillet, warm the corn tortillas over medium heat for about 30 seconds on each side, until they are pliable and lightly toasted.

5. Break the cooked fish into bite-sized pieces. Place a portion of fish onto each tortilla, top with a generous amount of cabbage slaw, and add a slice of avocado if desired.

6. Serve and enjoy!

Cooking Tips:
- For a smoky flavor, grill the fish filets instead of cooking them in a skillet.
- If you prefer a spicier taco, add a pinch of cayenne pepper to the seasoning mixture or top with a few slices of fresh jalapeño.

Nutritional Information (per serving):
- Calories: 290
- Protein: 25g
- Carbohydrates: 20g
- Fiber: 5g
- Fat: 12g
- Sodium: 150mg
- Potassium: 600mg
- Phosphorus: 250mg

Beef Barley Soup

Prep Time: 15 minutes | Cook Time: 1 hour | Serves: 6

Ingredients:
- One lb lean beef stew meat, cut into small pieces
- 2 tablespoons olive oil
- 1 onion, chopped
- 2 cloves garlic, minced
- 2 carrots, diced
- 2 celery stalks, diced
- One cup of mushrooms, sliced
- 1/2 cup pearl barley
- 6 cups low-sodium beef broth
- 1 teaspoon dried thyme
- 1 teaspoon dried rosemary
- 1/2 teaspoon ground black pepper
- 1 bay leaf
- Two tablespoons fresh parsley, chopped

Instructions:

1. Warm up the olive oil in a big pot or dutch oven over medium heat. Add the beef stew meat and simmer for 5 to 7 minutes, or until browned all over. After taking the steak out of the saucepan, set it aside.

2. Stir in the diced carrots, minced garlic, chopped onion, diced celery and sliced mushroom cooking for another 5 minutes until they begin to soften.

3. Stir in the pearl barley and return the beef to the pot. Pour in the low-sodium beef broth and add the dried thyme, dried rosemary, ground black pepper, and bay leaf. Boil the mixture

4. Once the soup reaches a simmer, reduce the heat to low and cover the pot partially with a lid. Let the soup simmer gently for 45 minutes to 1 hour, stirring occasionally until the beef and barley are tender.

5. Remove the bay leaf and stir in the chopped fresh parsley. Taste and adjust seasoning if needed. Serve hot

Curried Shrimp Salad Rolls

Prep Time: 20 minutes | Cook Time: 10 minutes | Serves: 4

Ingredients:
- One lb shrimp, deveined
- 1 tablespoon olive oil
- 1 teaspoon curry powder
- 1/2 teaspoon ground black pepper
- 8 rice paper wrappers
- 1 cup shredded lettuce
- 1/2 cup shredded carrots
- 1/2 cucumber, julienned
- 1/4 cup fresh cilantro, chopped

Dressing:
- 1/4 cup plain Greek yogurt
- 1 tablespoon lime juice
- 1/2 teaspoon curry powder
- 1 teaspoon honey

Instructions:
1. Warm olive oil over medium-high heat. Add the black pepper, curry powder, and shrimp. Cook until the shrimp are opaque and pink, 3 to 4 minutes. Take off the heat source and leave it to cool.

2. Whisk together the plain Greek yogurt, lime juice, curry powder, and honey in a bowl until smooth. Set aside.

3. On a cutting board, prepare the shredded lettuce, shredded carrots, and julienned cucumber. Have the chopped cilantro ready.

4. Fill a large shallow dish with warm water. Dip one rice paper wrapper into the water for about 10-15 seconds, or until it softens. On a spotless surface, place the softened wrapper flat

5. Place a small amount of lettuce, carrots, cucumber, and cilantro in the center of the wrapper. Add a few shrimp on top. Drizzle a small amount of the curry dressing over the filling.

6. Fold the bottom of the wrapper over the filling, then fold in the sides, and roll tightly to close. Continue with the remaining wrappers and filling.

7. Arrange the rolls on a serving platter. Serve immediately with any remaining curry dressing on the side for dipping.

Serving Suggestions:
- Pair the Curried Shrimp Salad Rolls with a light vegetable soup or a side of steamed edamame for a balanced meal.

Cooking Tips:
- To save time, use pre-cooked shrimp and simply toss with the curry powder and black pepper.
- For added crunch, include thinly sliced bell peppers or radishes in the rolls.

Nutritional Information (per serving):
- Calories: 220
- Protein: 20g
- Carbohydrates: 20g
- Fiber: 3g
- Fat: 8g
- Sodium: 150mg
- Potassium: 400mg
- Phosphorus: 150mg

Pasta Salad with Red Pepper Sauce

Prep Time: 20 minutes | Cook Time: 15 minutes | Serves: 4

Ingredients:
- Eight oz of whole wheat pasta (such as fusilli or penne)
- 1 big red bell pepper
- 1 tablespoon olive oil
- 1/2 cup plain Greek yogurt
- 1 clove garlic, minced
- 1 tablespoon fresh lemon juice
- 1 teaspoon dried basil
- 1/2 teaspoon ground black pepper
- 1/2 cup cherry tomatoes, halved
- 1/2 cucumber, diced
- 1/4 cup red onion, finely chopped
- 2 tablespoons fresh parsley, chopped

Instructions:
1. Heat up a big saucepan of water until it boils. When the pasta is al dente, add the whole wheat spaghetti and cook it as directed on the package. Rinse with cold water to allow it to cool down, keep aside.

2. Turn the oven on to 400°F (200°C) while the pasta cooks. After placing the red bell pepper on a baking sheet, roast it for about 20 minutes, rotating it halfway through, until the skin becomes blistered and roasted. Take out of the oven, transfer to a basin, and steam for ten minutes covered with plastic wrap. Chop the pepper, remove the seeds, and peel the skin.

3. Place the chopped red pepper, olive oil, plain Greek yogurt, minced garlic, lemon juice, dried basil, and ground black pepper in a blender or food processor.

4. Mix the cooked pasta, halved cherry tomatoes, diced cucumber, finely chopped red onion, and fresh parsley in a large bowl. Pour the red pepper sauce over the pasta and vegetables. Stir it to make sure it is mixed evenly.

5. Serve immediately, or refrigerate for 30 minutes to allow the flavors to combine well.

Serving Suggestions:
- Pair this pasta salad with a simple grilled chicken breast or fish filet for added protein.
- Serve alongside a mixed green salad with a light vinaigrette for a complete meal.
- Enjoy with a slice of whole grain bread or a small side of fruit for a refreshing contrast.

Cooking Tips:
- For a smoky flavor, you can grill the red pepper instead of roasting it.
- Add a handful of baby spinach or arugula for extra greens and a pop of color.
- Leftovers can be stored in an airtight container in the refrigerator for up to two days. Toss gently before serving.

Nutritional Information (per serving):
- Calories: 280
- Protein: 10g
- Carbohydrates: 42g
- Fiber: 7g
- Fat: 9g
- Sodium: 120mg
- Potassium: 450mg
- Phosphorus: 150mg

Shrimp and Apple Stir-Fry

Prep Time: 15 minutes | Cook Time: 10 minutes | Serves: 4

Ingredients:
- One lb shrimp, peeled and deveined
- 2 tablespoons olive oil
- 1 apple, thinly sliced (such as Granny Smith or Fuji)
- 1 red bell pepper
- 1 cup snap peas
- 1 carrot, julienned

- 2 cloves garlic, minced
- 1 teaspoon fresh ginger, minced
- Two tablespoons low-sodium soy sauce
- 1 tablespoon honey
- 1 tablespoon apple cider vinegar
- 1/4 teaspoon ground black pepper
- Two tablespoons fresh cilantro, chopped (optional)

Instructions:

1. Combine the apple cider vinegar, honey, ground black pepper, and low-sodium soy sauce in a small mixing bowl. Put aside.

2. In a large pan or wok, heat 1 tablespoon of olive oil over medium-high heat. When the shrimp turn pink and opaque, add them and simmer for another two to three minutes. After taking the shrimp out of the pan, set it aside.

3. Add the last tablespoon of olive oil to the same skillet. Add the fresh ginger and minced garlic, and sauté for 30 seconds or so, or until fragrant. Add the carrot, snap peas, red bell pepper, and apple slices. Stir-fry the veggies for 3–4 minutes, or until they are crisp-tender.

4. Put the cooked shrimp back in the skillet. Cover the shrimp and veggies with the prepared sauce. Mix everything together and cook for a further one to two minutes, or until well cooked and coated.

5. Transfer the stir-fry to serving plates. Garnish with fresh cilantro if desired. Serve immediately.

Cooking Tips:
- If you prefer a bit of heat, sprinkle a pinch of red pepper flakes into the stir-fry.
- Leftovers can be stored in an airtight container in the refrigerator for up to two days.

Nutritional Information (per serving):
- Calories: 250
- Protein: 22g
- Carbohydrates: 20g
- Fiber: 4g
- Fat: 10g
- Sodium: 200mg
- Potassium: 500mg

- Phosphorus: 220mg

Chicken Lasagna with White Sauce:

Prep Time: 30 minutes | Cook Time: 45 minutes | Serves: 6

Ingredients:
- 9 lasagna noodles (whole wheat, if available)
- 2 cups cooked chicken breast, shredded
- 2 tablespoons olive oil
- 1 onion, finely chopped
- 2 cloves garlic, minced
- 1 cup ricotta cheese
- One cup of shredded mozzarella cheese
- 1/4 cup grated Parmesan cheese (low-sodium)
- Two cups of low-sodium chicken broth
- 1 cup unsweetened almond milk
- Three teaspoons of all-purpose flour
- 1/4 teaspoon ground nutmeg
- 1/4 teaspoon of ground black pepper
- 1 tablespoon fresh parsley, chopped (optional)

Instructions:
1. Heat up a big saucepan of water until it boils. Cook lasagna noodles according to package directions until al dente. To avoid sticking, drain and rinse under cold water. Put aside.

2. Heat two tablespoons of olive oil in a medium skillet over medium heat. When the garlic is aromatic, add the minced garlic and simmer for about 30 seconds. Stir in all-purpose flour and fry until just starting to turn golden, one to two minutes. Whisk continuously to prevent lumps as you gradually add the unsweetened almond milk and low-sodium chicken broth. Simmer for a further five minutes or until the sauce thickens. Add the ground black pepper and nutmeg and stir. Take off the heat and place aside.

3. Heat one tablespoon of olive oil in a big pan over medium heat. Add the finely chopped onion and cook for about 5 minutes, or until softened. Cook until well heated, stirring in the cooked chicken shreds. Take off the heat.

4. Turn the oven on to 375°F, or 190°C. Place the ricotta cheese and half of the made white sauce in a mixing bowl. Grease a 9 x 13-inch baking dish from bottom to top with a thin coating of white sauce.

5. Top with three lasagna noodles. Partially cover the noodles with half of the ricotta mixture and then half of the chicken and onion mixture. Add a half-cup of shredded mozzarella cheese on top.

6. Add three more noodles, the leftover ricotta mixture, and the leftover chicken mixture to the layers and repeat. Add the last three noodles and the leftover white sauce on top. Add the leftover mozzarella cheese and the grated Parmesan cheese on top.

7. Bake the baking dish for 25 minutes in a preheated oven covered with aluminum foil. After taking off the foil, bake for a further 20 minutes, or until the top is bubbling and brown.

8. Take the lasagna out of the oven, then let it for ten minutes before slicing. Garnish with fresh parsley, if preferred.

Serving Suggestions:
- Pair this Chicken Lasagna with a side of steamed green beans or a simple garden salad with a light vinaigrette.
- Enjoy with a slice of whole grain garlic bread for a complete meal.
- Completed with a small serving of fresh fruit for dessert.

Nutritional Information (per serving):
- Calories: 350
- Protein: 28g
- Carbohydrates: 30g
- Fiber: 3g
- Fat: 14g
- Sodium: 220mg
- Potassium: 450mg
- Phosphorus: 240mg

Shrimp Salad with Cucumber and Mint

Prep Time: 15 minutes | Cook Time: 10 minutes | Serves: 4

Ingredients:
- One lb shrimp, deveined
- 2 tablespoons olive oil
- 1 large cucumber, thinly sliced
- One quarter cup of red onion, sliced thinly
- One quarter cup of mint leaves, chopped
- 2 tablespoons fresh lemon juice
- 1 tablespoon apple cider vinegar
- 1 teaspoon honey
- 1/4 teaspoon of ground black pepper
- 1 tablespoon fresh dill, chopped (optional)

Instructions:

1. A medium pan filled with one tablespoon of olive oil is heated to medium-high heat. When the shrimp turn pink and opaque, add them and fry for two to three minutes on each side. After turning off the heat, give it some time to cool.

2. Whisk the lemon juice, honey, apple cider vinegar, and remaining 1 tablespoon olive oil together in a bowl. Mix thoroughly after adding the ground black pepper. Put aside.

3. Combine the chopped mint leaves, red onion, and cucumber slices in a large salad dish. To the bowl, add the shrimp.

4. Drizzle the salad with the dressing and gently toss to coat all the ingredients equally.

5. If desired, Garnish with fresh dill. Serve immediately.

Serving Suggestions:
- Pair this Shrimp Salad with a side of steamed asparagus or roasted bell peppers for a complete meal.
- Enjoy with a slice of whole grain bread or a small serving of quinoa for added fiber and nutrients.

Nutritional Information (per serving):

- Calories: 200
- Protein: 22g
- Carbohydrates: 10g
- Fiber: 2g
- Fat: 9g
- Sodium: 180mg
- Potassium: 400mg
- Phosphorus: 180mg

Tuna Rice Casserole

Prep Time: 20 minutes | Cook Time: 30 minutes | Serves: 6

Ingredients:

- 1 1/2 cups of cooked brown rice
- Two cans (5 oz each) of low-sodium tuna, drained
- 1 tablespoon olive oil
- 1 small onion, finely chopped
- 1 cup frozen peas and carrots, thawed
- One cup of almond milk, unsweetened
- 1/2 cup of chicken broth(low sodium)
- Two tablespoons of all-purpose flour
- 1/4 teaspoon ground black pepper
- 1/4 teaspoon dried thyme
- 1/2 cup of shredded mozzarella cheese (low sodium)
- 1/4 cup grated Parmesan cheese (low-sodium)
- 1 tablespoon fresh parsley, chopped (optional)

Instructions:

1. Turn the oven on to 375°F, or 190°C.

2. A medium pan filled with one tablespoon of olive oil is heated to medium-high heat. Add the finely chopped onion and cook for about 5 minutes, or until softened. After adding the carrots and thawed peas, simmer for a further three minutes.

3. Over medium heat, mix together the low-sodium chicken broth and almond milk in a medium saucepan. In order to prevent lumps, gradually whisk in the all-purpose flour while whisking continuously. Simmer for a further five minutes or until the sauce thickens. Add the dried thyme and ground black pepper and stir.

4. Transfer the cooked brown rice, drained tuna, sautéed veggies, and thickened sauce into a large mixing dish. To make sure everything is covered equally, thoroughly mix.

5. Spoon mixture into a 9 x 13-inch baking dish that has been buttered. Evenly distribute it. Top with a sprinkle of grated Parmesan and shredded mozzarella cheese.

6. Bake the casserole for 25 to 30 minutes, or until the top is bubbling and brown. Place the dish in the preheated oven.

7. Take the casserole out of the oven, and allow it to cool for approximately five minutes before serving.

Cooking Tips:
- If you prefer a creamier texture, add a bit more almond milk to the sauce.

Nutritional Information (per serving):
- Calories: 300
- Protein: 20g
- Carbohydrates: 30g
- Fiber: 4g
- Fat: 10g
- Sodium: 180mg
- Potassium: 420mg
- Phosphorus: 200mg

Peppered Chicken with Garlic and Honey

Prep Time: 15 minutes | Cook Time: 25 minutes | Serves: 4

Ingredients:
- 1 1/2 lbs of chicken breast, cut into strips
- 2 tablespoons olive oil

- 4 cloves garlic, minced
- 1/4 cup honey
- One tablespoon of low-sodium soy sauce
- 1/2 teaspoon of ground black pepper
- 1/4 teaspoon ground red pepper (optional, for heat)
- One tablespoon fresh parsley, chopped (optional)

Instructions:

1. Ground black pepper and, for added spiciness, a dash of ground red pepper are used to season the chicken strips.

2. Fill a big pan with one tablespoon of olive oil and heat it over medium-high heat. Add the chicken strips and heat, stirring periodically, for 5 to 7 minutes, or until cooked through and golden brown. Remove from the pan and put aside the chicken

3. Add the last tablespoon of olive oil to the same skillet. Add the minced garlic and lower the heat to medium. Take care not to burn the garlic while you sauté it for approximately 1 minute, just until aromatic.

4. Combine the low-sodium soy sauce and honey in a small mixing dish. Stirring to blend, pour the mixture into the skillet with the garlic. Cook for 2-3 minutes, allowing the sauce to thicken a little.

5. Return the cooked chicken to the skillet, tossing to coat it evenly with the garlic honey sauce. After the chicken is well cooked and well-glazed, cook it for a further two to three minutes.

Serving Suggestions:
- Pair this Peppered Chicken with a side of steamed broccoli or sautéed green beans for a balanced meal.
- Enjoy with a serving of brown rice or quinoa to complement the flavors.

Cooking Tips:
- For extra flavor, marinate the chicken strips in a bit of the honey and soy sauce mixture for 30 minutes before cooking.
- If you prefer a thicker sauce, allow it to simmer a bit longer until it reaches the desired consistency.

Nutritional Information (per serving):

- Calories: 350
- Protein: 30g
- Carbohydrates: 25g
- Fiber: 1g
- Fat: 12g
- Sodium: 200mg
- Potassium: 450mg
- Phosphorus: 230mg

Roasted Cauliflower with Rosemary

Prep Time: 10 minutes | Cook Time: 30 minutes | Serves: 4

Ingredients:
- One head of cauliflower, cut into florets
- 2 tablespoons olive oil
- 3 cloves garlic, minced
- 2 teaspoons fresh rosemary, chopped
- 1/4 teaspoon ground black pepper
- 1/2 lemon, juiced
- 1 tablespoon fresh parsley, chopped (optional)

Instructions:
1. Set oven temperature to 400°F, or 200°C. Line a baking sheet with parchment paper to make cleaning easier.

2. Place the cauliflower florets, olive oil, chopped rosemary, minced garlic, and ground black pepper in a large mixing basin. Make sure the oil and spices are properly distributed over the cauliflower by giving it a good toss.

3. Arrange the seasoned cauliflower florets on the baking pan in a single layer. Roast the cauliflower for 25 to 30 minutes in a preheated oven, tossing occasionally to ensure equal roasting, or until it is soft and golden brown.

4. Take the roasted cauliflower out of the oven and pour some freshly squeezed lemon juice over it. Toss gently to evenly distribute the lemon juice over the cauliflower.

5. If desired, garnish with fresh parsley and serve warm.

Serving Suggestions:
- Pair this roasted cauliflower with a quinoa salad or a bowl of lentil soup for a complete vegan meal.
- Serve alongside a main course of grilled vegetables or a vegan burger.

Nutritional Information (per serving):

- Calories: 90
- Protein: 2g
- Carbohydrates: 8g
- Fiber: 3g
- Fat: 6g
- Sodium: 20mg
- Potassium: 300mg
- Phosphorus: 40mg

Triple Berry Salad with Cottage Cheese

Prep Time: 15 minutes | Serves: 4

Ingredients:

- One cup of fresh strawberries, sliced
- One cup of fresh blueberries
- One cup of fresh raspberries
- One quarter cup of mint leaves, chopped
- One cup of cottage cheese(low sodium)
- Two tablespoon of honey (optional)
- 1 tablespoon lemon juice
- 1/2 teaspoon lemon zest

Instructions:

1. Sliced raspberries, blueberries, and strawberries should all be combined in a big mixing dish. Toss gently to properly distribute the berries.

2. Gently toss in the chopped mint leaves to evenly distribute them over the salad after adding them to the fruit mixture.

3. Combine the low-sodium cottage cheese, lemon juice, zest, and honey (if using) in a small mixing dish. Mix well to combine the flavors.

4. Distribute the berry mixture among four dishes for serving. Place a heaping tablespoon of the cottage cheese mixture on top of each serving.

Cooking Tips:

- For a vegan version, substitute the cottage cheese with a dairy-free alternative, such as almond or coconut milk yogurt.

Nutritional Information (per serving):

- Calories: 100
- Protein: 6g
- Carbohydrates: 18g
- Fiber: 4g
- Fat: 2g
- Sodium: 50mg
- Potassium: 220mg
- Phosphorus: 80mg

Asparagus Quiche

Prep Time: 20 minutes | Cook Time: 40 minutes | Serves: 6

Ingredients:
- One premade pie crust (check for low sodium options)
- One bunch of asparagus, cut into 1-inch pieces
- One small onion, chopped
- Two cloves of garlic, minced
- 1 tablespoon of olive oil
- Four eggs(egg whites)
- One cup of almond milk, unsweetened
- Half cup of shredded Swiss cheese (optional, reduce for lower protein)
- 1/4 teaspoon ground black pepper
- 1/4 teaspoon ground nutmeg
- 1 tablespoon fresh dill, chopped (optional)

Instructions:

1. Turn the oven on to 375°F, or 190°C. The pie dough should be put in a pie plate and left aside.

2. Fill a big pan with one tablespoon of olive oil and heat it over medium-high heat. Add the finely chopped onion and cook for 3–4 minutes, or until softened. One more minute is spent cooking after adding the minced garlic. Cook the asparagus pieces for a further five minutes, or until they are crisp-tender. After turning off the heat, give it some time to cool

3. In a mixing bowl, thoroughly mix the eggs, unsweetened almond milk, grated nutmeg, and ground black pepper.

4. Evenly distribute the sautéed veggies across the pie crust. If using, scatter the shredded Swiss cheese on top of the veggies. Make sure all of the veggies are covered when you pour the egg mixture over the top.

5. After the oven has been warmed, put the quiche inside and bake for 35 to 40 minutes, or until the filling is set and the top is browned. A knife put in the middle ought to emerge clean.

6. Before slicing, let the quiche cool for five to ten minutes. If preferred, garnish with fresh dill and serve warm.

Cooking Tips:
- To ensure the pie crust doesn't get soggy, pre-bake it for 10 minutes before adding the filling.
- For a richer flavor, substitute half of the almond milk with a low-sodium vegetable broth.

Nutritional Information (per serving):
- Calories: 180
- Protein: 9g
- Carbohydrates: 15g
- Fiber: 2g
- Fat: 10g
- Sodium: 120mg
- Potassium: 250mg
- Phosphorus: 130mg

Garlic Green Bean Salad

Prep Time: 15 minutes | Cook Time: 10 minutes | Serves: 4

Ingredients:
- One pound of fresh green beans, cut into 2-inch pieces
- 2 tablespoons olive oil
- Three cloves of garlic, sliced thinly
- 1 small red onion, sliced thinly
- 1/4 teaspoon ground black pepper
- 2 tablespoons lemon juice
- One teaspoon of fresh parsley, chopped
- 1/4 cup of slivered almonds, lightly toasted

Instructions:
1. Heat up a big saucepan of water until it boils. When the green beans are crisp-tender, add them and simmer for three to five minutes. To cease cooking, drain and rinse with cold water right away. Put aside.

2. Fill a big pan with one tablespoon of olive oil and heat it over medium-high heat. Add the thinly sliced garlic and cook for approximately two minutes, or until aromatic and golden brown. Add the sliced red onion and simmer for 3–4 minutes, or until softened.

3. Combine the cooked green beans, ground black pepper, lemon juice, and sautéed onions and garlic in a large mixing dish. Toss to distribute the seasonings evenly over the green beans.

4. Top the salad with toasted slivered almonds and chopped fresh parsley. Gently toss to combine.

Serving Suggestions:
- Pair this salad with a quinoa pilaf or a hearty lentil soup for a complete vegan meal.
- Serve as a side dish alongside grilled vegetables or a vegan burger.

Nutritional Information (per serving):
- Calories: 130

- Protein: 3g
- Carbohydrates: 10g
- Fiber: 4g
- Fat: 9g
- Sodium: 10mg
- Potassium: 250mg
- Phosphorus: 40mg

Tofu and Veggie Frittata

Prep Time: 15 minutes | Cook Time: 30 minutes | Serves: 4

Ingredients:
- One block (14 oz) of drained and crumbled firm tofu,
 - 1 small zucchini, diced
- One red bell pepper, diced
- 1 small onion, chopped
- 2 cloves of garlic, minced
- 2 tablespoons of olive oil
- 1 teaspoon of turmeric
- Half teaspoon of ground black pepper
- One quarter teaspoon red pepper flakes (optional)
- One cup of fresh spinach, chopped
- 1 tablespoon nutritional yeast
- 1/4 cup almond milk(unsweetened)
- 1/4 cup fresh basil, chopped (optional)

Instructions:
1. Turn the oven on to 375°F, or 190°C.

2. One tablespoon of olive oil should be heated over medium heat in a big skillet. Add the finely chopped onion and minced garlic, and cook for approximately 3 minutes, or until the onion becomes transparent. Cook for a further five minutes, or until the veggies are soft, after adding the diced zucchini and red bell pepper.

3. Combine the crumbled tofu, nutritional yeast, chopped fresh spinach, ground black pepper, turmeric, and red pepper flakes (if using) in a medium-sized mixing dish. Toss to blend thoroughly.

4. Stir everything together until the tofu mixture is uniformly spread after adding the sautéed veggies. In the skillet, warm up the 5 1 tablespoon of olive oil over medium heat. After adding the tofu and veggie combination to the pan, heat it for around 5 minutes, stirring occasionally, until the mixture is heated through and slightly firm.

5. Spoon the batter into a 9-inch baking dish that has been gently oiled. Using a spatula, level the top and bake for 20 to 25 minutes, or until the frittata is set and has a light golden crust.

6. Take it out of the oven and give it some time to cool. Add freshly chopped basil as a garnish. Cut into pieces and reheat up.

Cooking Tips:
- Ensure the tofu is well-drained and crumbled to achieve the best texture.
- Feel free to add other low-potassium vegetables like mushrooms or bell peppers to the frittata.

Nutritional Information (per serving):
- Calories: 180
- Protein: 10g
- Carbohydrates: 10g
- Fiber: 3g
- Fat: 12g
- Sodium: 25mg
- Potassium: 250mg
- Phosphorus: 90mg

Eggplant and Chickpea Bites

Prep Time: 15 minutes | Cook Time: 25 minutes | Serves: 4

Ingredients:
- One medium of eggplant, diced
- One can (15 oz) of rinsed and drained chickpeas

- 1 small onion, chopped
- 2 cloves garlic, minced
- 2 tablespoons olive oil
- 1 teaspoon ground cumin
- 1/2 teaspoon smoked paprika
- 1/4 teaspoon ground black pepper
- 1/4 cup fresh parsley, chopped
- 2 tablespoons lemon juice
- 1/4 cup breadcrumbs (use gluten-free if needed)

Instructions:

1. Turn the oven on to 375°F, or 190°C. Use parchment paper to line a baking sheet.

2. Transfer the diced eggplant to the baking sheet that has been ready. Pour one tablespoon of olive oil over it and toss to coat. Roast for 15 minutes, or until tender, in a preheated oven.

3. In a pan over medium heat, warm up 1 tablespoon of olive oil while the eggplant roasts. Add the finely chopped onion and cook for about 5 minutes, or until softened. When the garlic is aromatic, add the minced garlic and simmer for a further one to two minutes.

4. Place the roasted eggplant, drained chickpeas, sautéed onion and garlic, ground cumin, smoked paprika, ground black pepper, fresh parsley, and lemon juice in a food processor or blender. Pulse the mixture until it is thoroughly mixed but still still slightly chunky.

5. Move the blend into a spacious mixing basin and blend in the breadcrumbs. Shape the mixture into 1-2 inch-diameter bite-sized or patties.

6. Transfer the bites to the parchment paper-lined baking sheet. Preheat the oven to 200°C. Bake for 20 minutes, rotating the dish halfway through, or until the outside is crispy and golden brown. Savor hot or room temperature.

Nutritional Information (per serving):
- Calories: 150
- Protein: 5g
- Carbohydrates: 20g
- Fiber: 6g

- Fat: 6g
- Sodium: 40mg
- Potassium: 350mg
- Phosphorus: 90mg

Turnip Greens and Sautéed Kale

Prep Time: 10 minutes | Cook Time: 15 minutes | Serves: 4

Ingredients:
- One bunch of kale, chopped
- One bunch turnip greens, chopped
- 2 tablespoons of olive oil
- Three cloves of garlic, minced
- 1 small onion, finely chopped
- One quarter teaspoon of ground black pepper
- One quarter teaspoon of red pepper flakes (optional)
- One tablespoon of fresh lemon juice

Instructions:
1. Thoroughly wash the turnip and kale greens. After trimming off any rough stems, cut the leaves into small pieces.

2. Warm up the olive oil in a large pan over medium heat. Add the finely chopped onion and sauté for around three minutes once the onion has softened. Add the minced garlic and cook for one more minute once it becomes fragrant.

3. Stir the chopped turnip greens and kale into the pan with the onions and garlic. Cook, tossing occasionally, until the greens are soft and wilted, approximately 5 to 7 minutes.

4. Top the greens with a sprinkle of red pepper flakes (if using) and ground black pepper. To evenly spread the seasoning, stir. Simmer for a further two minutes.

5. Turn off the heat and pour in the freshly lemon juice over the greens. Mix them together

Nutritional Information (per serving):
- Calories: 120
- Protein: 4g
- Carbohydrates: 10g
- Fiber: 4g
- Fat: 8g
- Sodium: 30mg
- Potassium: 500mg
- Phosphorus: 50mg

Hearty Mashed Potatoes

Prep Time: 15 minutes | Cook Time: 20 minutes | Serves: 4

Ingredients:
- Four russet potatoes, peeled and cut into large pieces
- One quarter cup of almond milk(unsweetened)
- Two tablespoons of unsalted butter
- One quarter teaspoon of garlic powder
- One quarter teaspoon of ground black pepper
- 1/4 teaspoon of dried thyme
- One tablespoon of chives, chopped (optional)

Instructions:

1. Put the potatoes in a big saucepan, chunked and skinned. Over medium-high heat, cover with cold water and bring to a boil. Lower the heat to a simmer and continue cooking for 15 to 20 minutes, or until the potatoes are soft.

2. Transfer the potatoes back to the saucepan after draining them in a strainer. Once the potatoes are smooth and creamy, add the unsalted butter and mash.

3. Add the unsweetened almond milk little by little, stirring to get the right consistency. Stir in the dried thyme, powdered black pepper, and garlic powder.

4. Garnish with freshly chopped chives, if preferred, and serve hot.

- Calories: 180
- Protein: 4g
- Carbohydrates: 30g
- Fiber: 3g
- Fat: 6g
- Sodium: 25mg
- Potassium: 600mg
- Phosphorus: 60mg

Roasted Paprika Laced Cauliflower

Prep Time: 10 minutes | Cook Time: 25 minutes | Serves: 4

Ingredients:
- One head of cauliflower, cut into florets
- 2 tablespoons olive oil
- 1 teaspoon smoked paprika
- 1/2 teaspoon garlic powder
- 1/2 teaspoon ground cumin
- 1/4 teaspoon ground black pepper
- 1 tablespoon fresh lemon juice
- 2 tablespoons fresh parsley, chopped

Instructions:
1. Warm up your oven to 400°F, or 200°C.

2. Make sure every floret of cauliflower is fully coated by tossing it in a big dish of olive oil.

3. Dust the cauliflower with ground cumin, ground black pepper, smoked paprika, and garlic powder. Remix to ensure that the spices are dispersed equally.

The seasoned cauliflower florets should be arranged on a baking pan in a single layer. Stir the cauliflower midway through to promote equal cooking and roast for 20 to 25 minutes, or until it is soft and gently toasted.

5. Take out of the oven, then quickly pour some freshly squeezed lemon juice over the cauliflower. Cast aside to coat.

6. Place the cooked cauliflower on a platter and top with freshly cut parsley. Hot servings are recommended.

Nutritional Information (per serving):
- Calories: 120
- Protein: 3g
- Carbohydrates: 10g
- Fiber: 4g
- Fat: 8g
- Sodium: 50mg
- Potassium: 450mg
- Phosphorus: 50mg

Berry Tofu Smoothie

Prep Time: 5 minutes | Serves: 2

Ingredients:
- 1/2 cup of silken tofu
- One cup of almond milk (unsweetened)
- Half cup of fresh or frozen strawberries
- Half cup of blueberries(either fresh or frozen)
- One teaspoon of chia seeds
- One teaspoon of agave nectar (optional)
- Half teaspoon of vanilla extract
- A handful of ice cubes (optional)

Instructions:

1. In a blender, add the silken tofu, unsweetened almond milk, strawberries, blueberries, chia seeds, agave nectar (if using), and vanilla extract.

2. The mixture should be smooth and creamy after blending on high. For a thicker consistency, add a handful of ice cubes and blend again.

3. Pour the smoothie into glasses and enjoy immediately for the best flavor and texture.

Nutritional Information (per serving):
- Calories: 120
- Protein: 6g
- Carbohydrates: 18g
- Fiber: 4g
- Fat: 3g
- Sodium: 30mg
- Potassium: 180mg
- Phosphorus: 50mg

Rhubarb Lemonade Punch

Prep Time: 10 minutes | Cook Time: 20 minutes | Serves: 4

Ingredients:
- Two cups of chopped rhubarb
- Four cups of water
- 1/2 cup of fresh lemon juice
- Half quarter cup of honey or agave nectar
- Ice cubes

Instructions

1. Chop the rhubarb and add the water to a pot. Bring to a boil over medium heat, then lower to a simmer. Cook for about 15-20 minutes, until the rhubarb is tender and broken down.

2. Turn off the heat and let the pot take a little time to cool. Sift the rhubarb mixture into a large pitcher, pressing to remove as much liquid as possible from the solids. Throw out the solids.

3. Stir in the fresh lemon juice and honey or agave nectar until well combined. Adjust sweetness to taste.

4. Refrigerate the punch for at least an hour to chill thoroughly.

5. Fill glasses with ice cubes and pour the chilled rhubarb lemonade punch over the ice.

Nutritional Information (per serving):
- Calories: 50
- Protein: 0g
- Carbohydrates: 13g
- Fiber: 1g
- Fat: 0g
- Sodium: 10mg
- Potassium: 150mg
- Phosphorus: 15mg

Peach Raspberry Smoothie

Prep Time: 5 minutes | Serves: 2

Ingredients:
- One cup of almond milk (unsweetened)
- One cup of fresh or frozen peach slices
- Half cup of fresh or frozen raspberries
- 1/2 cup of plain Greek yogurt (optional for extra creaminess)
- One tablespoon of chia seeds
-One tablespoon of agave nectar/honey (optional)
- A handful of ice cubes (optional)

Instructions:

1. Combine the unsweetened almond milk, peach slices, raspberries, plain Greek yogurt (if using), chia seeds, and honey or agave nectar (if desired) in a blender.

2. The mixture should be smooth and creamy after blending on high. For a thicker smoothie, add a handful of ice cubes and blend again until smooth.

3. Pour the smoothie into glasses and enjoy immediately to appreciate its fresh flavors and creamy texture.

Nutritional Information (per serving):
- Calories: 130
- Protein: 3g
- Carbohydrates: 22g
- Fiber: 5g
- Fat: 3g
- Sodium: 45mg
- Potassium: 220mg
- Phosphorus: 55mg

Peach Iced Tea

Prep Time: 10 minutes | Cook Time: 15 minutes | Chill Time: 1 hour | Serves: 4

Ingredients:
- Two ripe peaches, sliced
- 4 cups of water
- Two black tea bags (caffeine-free if preferred)
- Two teaspoons of agave nectar/honey
- One teaspoon of fresh lemon juice
- Ice cubes

Instructions:
1. Combine the sliced peaches and 2 cups of water to a pot. Bring to a boil over medium heat, then lower to a simmer. Cook for about 10 minutes, until the peaches are soft and broken down.

2. Turn off the heat and let the pot take a little time to cool. Pour the peach mixture through a strainer into a large pitcher, pressing the solids to extract as much liquid as possible. Discard the solids.

3. In another saucepan, bring the remaining 2 cups of water to a boil. Add the tea bags when the boiled water has been taken down from heat. Let steep for 5 minutes, then remove the tea bags and allow the tea to cool.

4. Add the cooled tea to the pitcher with the peach syrup. Stir in the honey or agave nectar and fresh lemon juice until well combined. Adjust sweetness to taste.

5. Refrigerate the peach iced tea for at least an hour to chill thoroughly.

6. Fill glasses with ice cubes and pour the chilled peach iced tea over the ice.

Nutritional Information (per serving):
- Calories: 40
- Protein: 0g
- Carbohydrates: 10g
- Fiber: 0g
- Fat: 0g

- Sodium: 5mg
- Potassium: 90mg
- Phosphorus: 10mg

Carrot Ginger Juice

Prep Time: 10 minutes | Serves: 2

Ingredients:
- Four large carrots, chopped
- 1-inch piece of fresh ginger, sliced
- 1 cup of cold water
- One teaspoon of lemon juice (optional for extra zest)
- Ice cubes (optional)

Instructions:
1. Peel and chop the carrots and ginger into small pieces for easier blending.

2. If using a blender, combine the carrots, ginger, and cold water. Blend on high until smooth.

3. Pour the blended mixture through a fine mesh strainer or cheesecloth into a bowl, pressing to extract as much juice as possible. Save the pulp for a different purpose and discard it

4. Stir in the lemon juice for an added burst of flavor, if desired.

5. Pour the juice into glasses over ice cubes, if preferred, and enjoy immediately.

Nutritional Information (per serving):
- Calories: 50
- Protein: 1g
- Carbohydrates: 12g
- Fiber: 2g
- Fat: 0g
- Sodium: 50mg
- Potassium: 320mg
- Phosphorus: 25mg

Cranberry Mint Mocktail

Prep Time: 10 minutes | Serves: 4

Ingredients:
- Two cups of cranberry juice (unsweetened)
- One cup cold water
- 1/4 cup fresh lime juice
- Two teaspoons of honey or agave nectar
- Half quarter cup fresh mint leaves, plus extra for garnish
- Ice cubes
- Sparkling water (optional)

Instructions

1. In a pitcher, add the fresh mint leaves and honey or agave nectar. Use a muddler or wooden spoon to gently muddle the mint, releasing its oils and flavors.

2. Add the unsweetened cranberry juice, cold water, and fresh lime juice to the pitcher. Stir well to combine.

3. Fill glasses with ice cubes and pour the cranberry mint mixture over the ice.

4. For a fizzy version, top each glass with a splash of sparkling water.

5. Garnish each glass with extra mint leaves for a fresh touch.

Nutritional Information (per serving):
- Calories: 40
- Protein: 0g
- Carbohydrates: 11g
- Fiber: 0g
- Fat: 0g
- Sodium: 5mg
- Potassium: 35mg
- Phosphorus: 5mg

Strawberry Basil Water

Prep Time: 5 minutes | Chill Time: 1 hour | Serves: 4

Ingredients:
- One cup of fresh strawberries, sliced
- Half quarter cup of fresh basil leaves
- Four cups of cold water
- Ice cubes
- Strawberry slices and basil sprigs for garnish (optional)

Instructions:
1. In a pitcher, combine the sliced strawberries and fresh basil leaves.

2. Use a wooden spoon to gently muddle the strawberries and basil together, releasing their flavors.

3. Pour the cold water into the pitcher, covering the strawberries and basil.

4. To enable the flavors to mingle, put the pitcher in the fridge and let it there for at least an hour.

5. Fill glasses with ice cubes and pour the chilled Strawberry Basil Water over the ice.

6. Optionally, garnish each glass with a slice of strawberry and a sprig of basil for an extra touch of freshness.

Nutritional Information (per serving):
- Calories: 5
- Protein: 0g
- Carbohydrates: 1g
- Fiber: 0g
- Fat: 0g
- Sodium: 0mg
- Potassium: 20mg
- Phosphorus: 5mg

Strawberry Rhubarb Lemonade

Prep Time: 15 minutes | Cook Time: 20 minutes | Chill Time: 1 hour | Serves: 4

Ingredients:
- One cup of chopped rhubarb
- One cup of fresh strawberries, sliced
- Four cups of water
- Half cup of fresh lemon juice
- One quarter cup of agave nectar/honey
- Ice cubes

Instructions:
1. Combine the sliced strawberries, chopped rhubarb and 2 cups of water to a pot. Bring to a boil over medium heat, then lower to a simmer. Cook for about 15-20 minutes, until the fruit is soft and has released its juices

2. Turn off the heat and let the pot take a little time to cool. Pour the mixture through a strainer into a large pitcher, pressing the solids to extract as much liquid as possible. Discard the solids.

3. Stir in the fresh lemon juice and honey or agave nectar until well combined. Adjust sweetness to taste.

4. Incorporate the leftover two cups of water into the pitcher and mix thoroughly.

5. Refrigerate the lemonade for at least an hour to chill thoroughly.

6. Fill glasses with ice cubes and pour the chilled strawberry rhubarb lemonade over the ice.

Nutritional Information (per serving):
- Calories: 45
- Protein: 0g
- Carbohydrates: 12g
- Fiber: 1g
- Fat: 0g
- Sodium: 5mg

- Potassium: 100mg
- Phosphorus: 10mg

Lime and Mint Soda

Prep Time: 10 minutes | Serves: 4

Ingredients:
- One quarter cup of fresh lime juice (about 2-3 limes)
- Two tablespoons of agave nectar/ honey
- 1/4 cup of fresh mint leaves
- 4 cups of water
- Ice cubes
- Lime slices and mint sprigs for garnish

Instructions:
1. In a pitcher, add the fresh mint leaves and honey or agave nectar. Use a muddler or wooden spoon to gently muddle the mint, releasing its fragrant oils and flavors.

2. Pour in the fresh lime juice and stir well to combine with the muddled mint and sweetener.

3. Slowly add the sparkling water to the pitcher, stirring gently to mix.

4. Fill glasses with ice cubes and pour the lime and mint soda over the ice.

5. Garnish each glass with lime slices and mint sprigs for an extra touch of freshness. Serve immediately and enjoy the invigorating flavors.

Nutritional Information (per serving):
- Calories: 20
- Protein: 0g
- Carbohydrates: 5g
- Fiber: 0g
- Fat: 0g
- Sodium: 5mg
- Potassium: 15mg
- Phosphorus: 5mg

Tuna Spread

Prep Time: 10 minutes | Serves: 4

Ingredients:
- One can (5 ounces) of drained low-sodium tuna
- 1/4 cup of plain Greek yogurt (low sodium)
- One tablespoon of lemon juice
- One tablespoon of chopped fresh dill
- One teaspoon of Dijon mustard
- One celery stalk, chopped
- One quarter teaspoon of black pepper
- Optional: a pinch of salt

Instructions:
1. Use a fork to break up the drained tuna into tiny pieces in a mixing dish.

2. Fill the bowl with the Greek yogurt, lemon juice, celery, minced dill, Dijon mustard, and black pepper.

3. Until the tuna is evenly coated and the spread is creamy, fully combine all the ingredients.

4. Taste the spread and, if needed, adjust the seasoning. If you would like, add a small amount of salt, but not too much to keep it kidney-friendly.

5. Savor right away or store in the fridge until needed.

Nutritional Information (per serving):
- Calories: 60
- Protein: 10g
- Carbohydrates: 2g
- Fiber: 0g
- Fat: 1g
- Sodium: 100mg

- Potassium: 100mg
- Phosphorus: 80mg

Pineapple Coleslaw

Prep Time: 15 minutes | Serves: 4

Ingredients:
- Two cups of shredded green cabbage
- One cup of shredded red cabbage
- One cup of fresh pineapple, chopped
- One medium carrot, shredded
- 1/4 cup of plain Greek yogurt (low sodium)
- One tablespoon of apple cider vinegar
- 1 teaspoon honey
- One quarter teaspoon of black pepper
- Optional: a pinch of salt

Instructions:
1. Shredded carrot, shredded red cabbage, shredded green cabbage, and chopped pineapple should all be combined in a big mixing dish.

2. Combine the plain Greek yogurt, honey, apple cider vinegar, and black pepper in a small bowl. If desired, add a pinch of salt after tasting the dressing.

3. Drizzle the pineapple and cabbage combination with the dressing. Make sure the dressing coats everything evenly by giving it a good toss.

4. Cover the coleslaw and refrigerate for at least 30 minutes before serving for optimal results. This enables the tastes to combine.

5. After the coleslaw cools, toss it one last time and serve.

Nutritional Information (per serving):
- Calories: 50
- Protein: 2g
- Carbohydrates: 10g

- Fiber: 2g
- Fat: 0.5g
- Sodium: 30mg
- Potassium: 150mg
- Phosphorus: 40mg

Spiced Almonds and Cashews

Prep Time: 10 minutes | Cook Time: 15 minutes | Serves: 6

Ingredients:
- One cup of raw almonds(without salt)
- One cup of raw cashews(without salt)
- 1 tablespoon olive oil
- 1 teaspoon ground cumin
- One teaspoon of smoked paprika
- Half teaspoon of garlic powder
- Half quarter teaspoon of cayenne pepper (optional, for heat)
- Half quarter teaspoon of black pepper
- Optional: 1/4 teaspoon salt

Instructions:
1. Adjust the oven temperature to 350°F (175°C) and place parchment paper on a baking pan.

2. Place the cashews and almonds in a mixing basin. After drizzling the nuts with olive oil, toss to ensure uniform coating.

3. Fill the bowl with the smoked paprika, garlic powder, ground cumin, black pepper, and salt (if using). Toss one more to make sure the nuts get a good coating of the spice combination.

4. Arrange the seasoned nuts on the baking sheet that has been preheated in a single layer. Bake, tossing occasionally, for 10 to 15 minutes in a preheated oven or until the nuts are aromatic and brown.

5. Take the baking sheet out of the oven, allowing the nuts to cool fully. After the nuts have cooled, move them to an airtight container for storage.

Nutritional Information (per serving):
- Calories: 180
- Protein: 6g
- Carbohydrates: 7g
- Fiber: 3g
- Fat: 15g
- Sodium: 10mg
- Potassium: 200mg
- Phosphorus: 100mg

Pita Wedges

Prep Time: 10 minutes | Cook Time: 10 minutes | Serves: 4

Ingredients:
- Two whole wheat pitas
- 1 tablespoon of olive oil
- 1 teaspoon of dried oregano
- Half teaspoon of garlic powder
- Half quarter teaspoon of black pepper
- **Optional**: 1/4 teaspoon salt

Instructions:
1. Use paper liners to line the baking pan.

2. Cut each whole wheat pita into eight pieces. Place the wedges in a single layer on the baking sheet that has been prepared.

3. In a small dish, mix the olive oil, dried oregano, garlic powder, black pepper, and salt (if using). Using a pastry brush, lightly coat the pita wedges with the seasoned olive oil mixture.

4. Bake the pita wedges for 8 to 10 minutes, or until they are crispy and golden brown, after putting the baking sheet inside the preheated oven.

5. Remove the baking sheet from the oven and allow the pita wedges to cool slightly. Serve at room temperature or reheat.

Nutritional Information (per serving):
- Calories: 80
- Protein: 2g
- Carbohydrates: 12g
- Fiber: 2g
- Fat: 3g
- Sodium: 60mg
- Potassium: 50mg
- Phosphorus: 50mg

Fruit Salsa

Prep Time: 15 minutes | Serves: 4

Ingredients:
- One cup of diced pineapple
- One cup of diced strawberries
- One medium apple, diced
- One kiwi diced
- One tablespoon of fresh lime juice
- 1 teaspoon honey
- One tablespoon of chopped mint

Instructions:
1. Put the chopped pineapple, strawberries, apple, and kiwi in a large mixing dish.

2. Pour honey and lime juice over the fruit mixture. Make sure the fruit is covered evenly by giving it a little toss to mix.

3. Drizzle the fruit with the finely chopped fresh mint and gently mix again.

4. Cover the bowl, place it in the refrigerator, and let the fruit salsa sit for at least half an hour before serving for optimal taste.

5. You may serve the fruit salsa cold with whole grain pita chips or by itself.

Nutritional Information (per serving):
- Calories: 70
- Protein: 1g
- Carbohydrates: 18g
- Fiber: 3g
- Fat: 0g
- Sodium: 2mg
- Potassium: 120mg
- Phosphorus: 20mg

Cornbread Muffins

Prep Time: 10 minutes | Cook Time: 15 minutes | Serves: 12

Ingredients:
- One cup of cornmeal
- One cup of all-purpose flour
- One tablespoon of baking powder (low sodium if available)
- 1/4 cup of sugar
- 1/4 teaspoon of salt (optional)
- One cup of almond milk(unsweetened)
- 1/4 cup of unsalted butter, melted
- One egg, whisked

Instructions:
1. Set oven temperature to 400°F, or 200°C. Use paper liners to line the muffin pan, or gently oil each cup.

2. Combine the cornmeal, flour, baking powder, sugar, and salt (if using) in a large mixing basin. Mix well by stirring.

3. Combine the melted butter, beaten egg, and almond milk in another bowl.

4. Mix the wet mixture with the dry mixture. Don't overmix; instead, stir gently until just blended.

5. Evenly spoon batter into muffin tray, filling each cup approximately two-thirds of the way.

6. Bake the muffin pan for 15 minutes, or until a toothpick inserted into the middle of a muffin comes out clean, in the preheated oven.

7. Let cool the muffins in the tin for a few minutes before transferring them to a wire rack to cool completely.

Nutritional Information (per muffin):
- Calories: 120
- Protein: 2g
- Carbohydrates: 20g
- Fiber: 1g
- Fat: 4g
- Sodium: 80mg
- Potassium: 60mg
- Phosphorus: 50mg

Herbed Cream Cheese Toast

Prep Time: 10 minutes | Serves: 4

Ingredients:
- Four slices of low-sodium whole grain bread
- Four ounces of low-fat cream cheese, softened
- One tablespoon of fresh parsley, chopped
- One tablespoon fresh chives, chopped
- One teaspoon fresh dill, chopped
- Half Teaspoon of garlic powder
- Half quarter teaspoon of black pepper

Instructions:
1. Chop the dill, chives, and parsley finely. Put aside.

2. Put the melted cream cheese, chopped herbs, garlic powder, and black pepper in a mixing bowl. Mix until smooth and fully mixed.

3. Use a toaster or toaster oven to toast the bread pieces until they are crisp and golden brown.

4. Cover each piece of bread with a thick coating of the herbed cream cheese mixture using a spatula.

5. Serve the toasts right away after cutting them into quarters or half for convenient munching.

Nutritional Information (per serving):
- Calories: 120
- Protein: 4g
- Carbohydrates: 15g
- Fiber: 2g
- Fat: 5g
- Sodium: 100mg
- Potassium: 80mg
- Phosphorus: 50mg

Buttermilk Biscuits

Prep Time: 15 minutes | Cook Time: 12 minutes | Makes: 12 biscuits

Ingredients:
- 2 cups whole wheat pastry flour
- One tablespoon of baking powder (low sodium)
- Half teaspoon of baking soda
- One quarter teaspoon of salt
- 1/4 cup of butter(without salt), cold and cubed
- 3/4 cup of low-fat buttermilk

Instructions:
1. Set the oven temperature to 425°F (220°C). Use paper liners to line the baking sheet.

2. Using a big mixing basin, thoroughly mix the whole wheat pastry flour, baking soda, baking powder, and salt.

3. Combine the dry ingredients with the chilled, diced butter. To make the butter into coarse crumbs, cut it into the flour mixture using a pastry cutter or fork.

4. After adding the buttermilk to the flour mixture, whisk just until incorporated. Don't blend too much.

5. Transfer the dough to a surface that has been lightly floured. Knead dough a few times gently until dough comes together. Don't overwork the dough.

6. Roll out the dough to a thickness of approximately 1/2 inch with a rolling pin. Cut circles of dough with a drinking glass or biscuit cutter. With a little space between each, place the biscuits on the baking sheet that has been prepared.

7. Using a pastry brush, lightly coat the biscuit tops with buttermilk. Bake for 10 to 12 minutes, or until the biscuits are cooked through and golden brown, in a preheated oven.

8. Take out of the oven and place the biscuits on a wire rack to cool gently. Heat or serve at room temperature.

Serving Suggestions:
- Enjoy with a spread of low-sodium jam or honey for a sweet treat.
- Make breakfast sandwiches with scrambled eggs and low-fat cheese for a protein-packed snack.

Nutritional Information (per biscuit):
- Calories: 120
- Protein: 3g
- Carbohydrates: 18g
- Fiber: 2g
- Fat: 4g
- Sodium: 150mg
- Potassium: 90mg
- Phosphorus: 100mg

Cooking Tips:
- For extra flakiness, fold the dough over itself a couple of times before rolling it out.

- Make sure your butter is cold and firm before cutting it into the flour mixture.

DESSERT RECIPES

Lemon Sherbet

Prep Time: 15 minutes | Freeze Time: 4 hours | Serves: 6

Ingredients:
- One cup of squeezed lemon juice (about 4-5 lemons)
- 1 cup of water
- 1/2 cup of sugar
- One cup of almond or low-fat milk
- One teaspoon of lemon zest
- Mint leaves for garnish (optional)

Instructions:
1. Juice the lemons until you have 1 cup of lemon juice. Use a zester or grater to get 1 teaspoon of lemon zest. Set aside.

2. Combine the the water and sugar in a mixing bowl. Stir until the sugar is completely dissolved. This may take a few minutes.

3. Add the lemon juice, lemon zest, and milk to the sugar-water mixture. Whisk all ingredients together

4. Pour the mixture into a freezer-safe container. Place in the freezer for about 1 hour or until it starts to firm up around the edges.

5. After 1 hour, remove the container from the freezer. Use a whisk or fork to break up any ice crystals that have formed, then return the container to the freezer. Repeat this process every hour for 3 hours to ensure a smooth texture.

6. After the final mix, leave the sherbet in the freezer for another hour or until it's fully set and scoopable.

7. Scoop the lemon sherbet into bowls or cones. If desired, garnish with mint leaves

Nutritional Information (per serving):
- Calories: 80
- Protein: 2g
- Carbohydrates: 20g
- Fiber: 0g
- Fat: 1g
- Sodium: 30mg
- Potassium: 50mg
- Phosphorus: 40mg

Blueberry Whipped Pie

Prep Time: 20 minutes | Chill Time: 2 hours | Serves: 8

Ingredients:
- One prepared low-sodium graham cracker crust
- Two cups of blueberries
- Half cup of sugar
- 1 tablespoon of cornstarch
- 1/4 cup of water
- One teaspoon of lemon juice
- One teaspoon of lemon zest
- One cup of whipped topping (such as Cool Whip)
- Mint leaves for garnish (optional)

Instructions:
1. Combine the blueberries, sugar, cornstarch, and water. Stir well to mix.

2. Place the saucepan over medium heat. Cook, stirring frequently, until the mixture thickens and the blueberries begin to break down, about 10 minutes.

3. Remove the saucepan from heat and stir in the lemon juice and lemon zest. Allow the blueberry mixture to cool to room temperature.

4. In a mixing bowl, fold the whipped topping into the cooled blueberry mixture. Gently mix until well combined.

5. Spoon the blueberry and whipped topping mixture into the prepared graham cracker crust. Use a spatula to spread it flat

6. Place the pie in the refrigerator and chill for at least 2 hours, or until set.

7. If desired, garnish with mint leaves

Nutritional Information (per serving):
- Calories: 180
- Protein: 2g
- Carbohydrates: 30g
- Fiber: 2g
- Fat: 7g
- Sodium: 120mg
- Potassium: 60mg
- Phosphorus: 50mg

Baked Pear with Honey and Cinnamon

Prep Time: 10 minutes | Cook Time: 30 minutes | Serves: 4

Ingredients:
- Four ripe pears, sliced
- 2 tablespoons of honey
- 1 teaspoon of ground cinnamon
- 1/4 teaspoon of ground nutmeg (optional)
- 1/4 cup water
- Mint leaves for garnish (optional)

Instructions:
1. Set the oven temperature to 350°F (175°C).

2. After cleaning the pears, split them in half, and use a spoon to extract the cores. Place the pear halves in a baking dish, cut side up.

3. Combine the nutmeg (if using), honey, and cinnamon in a small bowl. Mix well by stirring.

4. Generously coat the sliced sides of the pears with the honey mixture using a basting brush. Fill the baking dish with water, around the pears.

5. Use foil to cover the baking dish. For about 25 to 30 minutes, or until the pears are soft and readily punctured with a fork, bake them in a preheated oven.

6. Remove the pears from the oven and let them cool slightly. Serve warm, If desired, garnished with mint leaves

Nutritional Information (per serving):
- Calories: 100
- Protein: 0.5g
- Carbohydrates: 25g
- Fiber: 4g
- Fat: 0g
- Sodium: 1mg
- Potassium: 150mg
- Phosphorus: 15mg

Ice Cream Pumpkin Pie

Prep Time: 20 minutes | Freeze Time: 4 hours | Serves: 8

Ingredients:
- One prepared low-sodium graham cracker crust
- One cup of pumpkin puree (canned or homemade)
- 1/2 cup of sugar
- 1 teaspoon of ground cinnamon
- Half teaspoon of ground ginger
- Half quarter teaspoon of ground nutmeg
- Half quarter teaspoon of ground cloves
- Two cups of low-fat vanilla ice cream (softened)

- Whipped topping for garnish (optional)
- Ground cinnamon for garnish (optional)

Instructions:
1. Combine the pumpkin puree, sugar, cinnamon, ginger, nutmeg, and cloves in a bowl. Whisk until the mixture is smooth and the spices are evenly distributed.

2. Gently fold the softened vanilla ice cream into the pumpkin mixture. Use a spatula to mix until well combined, ensuring a smooth consistency.

3. Spoon the pumpkin and ice cream mixture into the prepared graham cracker crust. Spread it flat with the spatula.

4. Cover the pie with plastic wrap and place it in the freezer for at least 4 hours, or until fully set.

5. Remove the pie from the freezer about 10 minutes before serving to allow it to soften slightly. Slice and serve with a dollop of whipped topping and a sprinkle of ground cinnamon if desired.

Nutritional Information (per serving):
- Calories: 180
- Protein: 3g
- Carbohydrates: 32g
- Fiber: 2g
- Fat: 5g
- Sodium: 120mg
- Potassium: 90mg
- Phosphorus: 60mg

Lemon Ricotta Cheesecake

Prep Time: 20 minutes | Cook Time: 50 minutes | Chill Time: 2 hours | Serves: 8

Ingredients:
- One prepared low-sodium graham cracker crust
- One cup of ricotta cheese
- Half cup of low-fat cream cheese, softened

- 1/2 cup of sugar
- Two eggs
- 1/4 cup of lemon juice
- One tablespoon of lemon zest
- One teaspoon of vanilla extract
- Fresh berries for garnish (optional)
- Fresh mint leaves for garnish (optional)

Instructions:
1. Set the oven temperature to 325°F (165°C).

2. In a mixing bowl, combine the ricotta cheese, low-fat cream cheese, and sugar. Blend until smooth, using a whisk or an electric mixer.

3. Beat thoroughly after adding each egg, one at a time. Add the vanilla essence, lemon zest, and lemon juice and stir until well combined.

4. Pour the lemon ricotta mixture into the prepared graham cracker crust, spreading it evenly with a spatula.

5. Place the springform pan in the preheated oven and bake for 45-50 minutes, or until the center is set and the top is lightly golden.

6. Remove the cheesecake from the oven and let it cool to room temperature. After cooling, place in the refrigerator to set for at least two hours.

7. Slice the cheesecake and serve chilled. If desired, garnish with fresh berries and mint leaves

Nutritional Information (per serving):
- Calories: 200
- Protein: 6g
- Carbohydrates: 25g
- Fiber: 0g
- Fat: 8g
- Sodium: 150mg
- Potassium: 90mg
- Phosphorus: 100mg

Sweet Mascarpone and Berries

Prep Time: 15 minutes | Serves: 4

Ingredients:
- One cup of mascarpone cheese
- Two tablespoons of honey
- One teaspoon of vanilla extract
- One cup of strawberries, hulled and halved
- One cup of blueberries
- One cup of raspberries
- Mint leaves for garnish (optional)

Instructions:
1. In a mixing bowl, combine the mascarpone cheese, honey, and vanilla extract. Blend until smooth and creamy using an electric mixer or

2. In serving glasses or bowls, add a layer of the mascarpone mixture. Top with a handful of strawberries, blueberries, and raspberries. Repeat the layers if desired.

3. Finish with a dollop of the mascarpone mixture on top. If desired, garnish with mint leaves

Nutritional Information (per serving):
- Calories: 220
- Protein: 4g
- Carbohydrates: 20g
- Fiber: 4g
- Fat: 14g
- Sodium: 20mg
- Potassium: 150mg
- Phosphorus: 70mg

Pumpkin Mousse Pie

Prep Time: 25 minutes | Chill Time: 4 hours | Serves: 8

Ingredients:
- One prepared low-sodium graham cracker crust
- One cup of pumpkin puree (canned or homemade)
- Half cup of sugar
- One teaspoon of ground cinnamon
- Half teaspoon of ground ginger
- Half quarter teaspoon of ground nutmeg
- Half quarter teaspoon of ground cloves
- One teaspoon of vanilla extract
- One cup heavy cream, chilled
- Half quarter cup of powdered sugar
- Whipped topping for garnish (optional)
- Ground cinnamon for garnish (optional)

Instructions:
1. In a mixing bowl, combine the pumpkin puree, sugar, ground cinnamon, ground ginger, ground nutmeg, ground cloves, and vanilla extract. Mix until smooth and the spices are evenly distributed.

2. In a separate bowl, whip the chilled heavy cream with the powdered sugar until stiff peaks form.

3. Gently fold the pumpkin mixture into the whipped cream using a spatula. Be careful not to deflate the whipped cream too much; you want to maintain the light, airy texture.

4. Spoon the pumpkin mousse into the prepared graham cracker crust, spreading it evenly with the spatula.

5. Cover the pie with plastic wrap and place it in the refrigerator for at least 4 hours to set.

6. Remove the pie from the refrigerator just before serving. Slice and serve with a dollop of whipped topping and a sprinkle of ground cinnamon if desired.

Nutritional Information (per serving):
- Calories: 230
- Protein: 3g
- Carbohydrates: 27g
- Fiber: 2g
- Fat: 14g
- Sodium: 120mg
- Potassium: 150mg
- Phosphorus: 80mg

Strawberry Brûlée

Prep Time: 10 minutes | Cook Time: 5 minutes | Serves: 4

Ingredients:
- Two cups of strawberries, hulled and halved
- 2 tablespoons of granulated sugar
- One teaspoon of vanilla extract
- One tablespoon of lemon juice
- Two tablespoons of brown sugar

Instructions:
1. Put the strawberries, lemon juice, vanilla essence, and granulated sugar in a mixing dish. To uniformly coat the strawberries, toss lightly.

2. Use paper liners to line the baking sheet. Arrange the strawberries on the sheet in a single layer.

3. Distribute the brown sugar evenly over the strawberries' surface. If necessary, use a tiny sieve to evenly distribute the sugar.

4. Using a kitchen torch, caramelize the brown sugar until it forms a crispy, golden crust. If you don't have a torch, place the baking sheet under the oven broiler on high for 2-3 minutes, watching closely to avoid burning.

5. Transfer the caramelized strawberries to serving bowls and enjoy immediately for the best texture and flavor.

Nutritional Information (per serving):
- Calories: 60
- Protein: 1g
- Carbohydrates: 14g
- Fiber: 2g
- Fat: 0g
- Sodium: 1mg
- Potassium: 140mg
- Phosphorus: 15mg

CONCLUSION

Taking care of your kidneys through a special diet might seem tough at first, but it's totally doable. By learning about how your kidneys work, understanding what foods are good for you, and using smart cooking tricks, you can make a big difference in your health. Remember, you're not alone in this journey. Your doctors and other people going through similar things are here to help. Stay positive, keep trying new things, and remember that every healthy choice you make is a step toward feeling better. Your health is in your hands, so let's give those kidneys the love and care they deserve!

<u>I Have A Request</u>

Dear Readers,

I hope you've been enjoying the delicious and healthful journey with my book, "Renal Diet Cookbook For Beginners." I've poured my heart and expertise into creating a resource that makes managing kidney disease simpler and more enjoyable for beginners.

Your feedback means the world to me! If you've had a chance to try out some of the recipes, I would be incredibly grateful if you could take a moment to share your thoughts. Your reviews not only help others who might be considering the book but also provide me with invaluable insights into how I can continue to serve you better.

Writing a review is easy and doesn't take long. You can share what you loved, your favorite recipes, or how this cookbook has made a difference in your daily routine. Every word you write is appreciated and helps to spread the word about living a healthier life with kidney disease.

Please leave your review in English on the platform where you purchased the book or on any book review sites. Thank you for your support, and I look forward to reading your experiences and success stories!

Warm regards,
[Kimberly Mullins]

To stay updated on my latest releases, events, and behind-the-scenes insights, please visit my Author Central page at [https://www.amazon.com/author/mullinskimberly]. Discover more about my passion for creating delectable recipes, hosting memorable gatherings, and nurturing a love for the culinary arts. Thank you for your support, and may your culinary journey continue to be filled with joy and delicious discoveries!

BONUS PAGE